Case Studies in General and Systematic Pathology

J.C.E. Underwood MD FRCPath

Joseph Hunter Professor of Pathology,
University of Sheffield Medical School;
Honorary Consultant Histopathologist,
Royal Hallamshire Hospital,
Sheffield

D.W.K. Cotton BSc PhD BM MD MRCPath

Reader in Pathology,
University of Sheffield Medical School;
Honorary Consultant Histopathologist,
Royal Hallamshire Hospital, Sheffield

S.S. Cross BSc MB BS MD MRCPath

Senior Lecturer,
Department of Pathology,
University of Sheffield Medical School;
Honorary Consultant Histopathologist,
Central Sheffield University Hospitals NHS Trust,
Sheffield

T.J. Stephenson MD MHSM MRCPath

Consultant Histopathologist,
Central Sheffield Hospitals Trust,
Sheffield

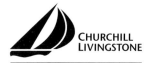

CHURCHILL
LIVINGSTONE

NEW YORK EDINBURGH LONDON MADRID MELBOURNE SAN FRANCISO AND TOKYO 1996

CHURCHILL LIVINGSTONE
Medical Division of Pearson Professional Limited

Distributed in the United States of America by Churchill Livingstone
Inc., 650 Avenue of the Americas, New York, N.Y. 10011, and by
associated companies, branches and representatives throughout the
world.

©Pearson Professional Limited 1996

First pubished 1996

ISBN 0 443 050961

British Library of Cataloguing in Publication Data
A catalogue record for this book is available from the British Library.

Library of Congress Cataloging in Publication Data
A catalog record for this book is available from the Library of Congress.

Printed in Hong Kong

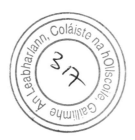

Preface

Most medical schools are adopting integrated curricula and encouraging problem-oriented learning. Pathology has a central role in all styles of medical curricula because it provides the scientific foundation for clinical practice. By integration with other disciplines, students can understand how clinical signs and symptoms provide clues to the underlying structural and functional obnormalities and, further, how knowledge of these abnormalities gives a rational basis for treatment. *Case Studies in General and Systematic Pathology*, a companion textbook to *General and Systematic Pathology* (2nd edition, Churchill Livingstone, 1996), edited by J.C.E. Underwood, and to the *MCQ Companion to General and Systematic Pathology* (2nd edition, Churchill Livingstone, 1996) by S.S. Cross, provides an integrated approach in the form of problem-oriented learning, enabling students to test their own knowledge and deductive skills.

The cases cover a wide range of problems and are based on actual clinical experiences. In each case, the clinical story is interrupted by a series of questions relevant to that point in the patient's history; the questions may be about the differential diagnosis, the disease mechanisms, the most appropriate investigations, or the interpretation of abnormal findings. We have illustrated not only the application of pathological principles to clinical problems in the living, but also the educational value of the autopsy. Revision boxes at the end of each case refer the reader to the relevant pages in *General and Systematic Pathology* for follow-up reading.

These case studies will provide students with interesting clinical scenarios on which to build their understanding of pathology and medicine.

Sheffield, 1996

J.C.E.U.
D.W.K.C.
S.S.C.
T.J.S.

Acknowledgements

The authors are grateful to Dr Andrew Messenger, Dr Michael Snaith and Dr David Winfield, for supplying some clinical photographs. Our radiological colleagues are acknowledged next to the illustrations they provided.

J.C.E.U.
D.W.K.C.
S.S.C.
T.J.S.

Contents

Diarrhoea

A 25-year-old female is seen urgently at the gastroenterology outpatient department at the request of her general practitioner. She complains of a sudden onset of bloody diarrhoea and abdominal pain. She has had no previous bouts of diarrhoea and her only significant past medical history was an episode of endocarditis of the tricuspid valve treated 2 years previously.

◆ **Question 1.1**
What processes may cause acute diarrhoea?

◆ **Question 1.2**
Why is the distinction between these two types of processes important?

The patient is admitted to the ward and rehydrated by intravenous fluids. The next day a flexible sigmoidoscopy is performed. The rectal and sigmoid mucosa is hyperaemic and some ulcers are visible. A biopsy is taken from the base of one of the ulcers and its histological appearances are shown in Figure 1.1.

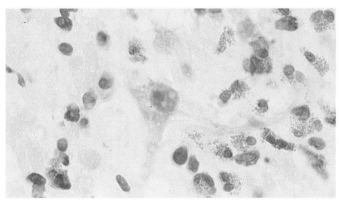

Fig. 1.1

◆ **Question 1.3**
What is present in the nucleus of the cell in the centre of the picture?

◆ **Question 1.4**
What infective agent may produce such objects?

The patient is treated with ganciclovir and over a week her symptoms settle.

◆ **Question 1.5**
What other investigations would you wish to carry out?

◆ **Answer 1.1**
Infective agents, commonly bacteria, may induce inflammation of the small and large bowel with subsequent diarrhoea. Inflammatory bowel disease, such as ulcerative colitis or Crohn's disease may also produce acute diarrhoea.

◆ **Answer 1.2**
Inflammatory bowel disease may be treated with anti-inflammatory agents such as steroids but these would worsen infective colitis by reducing the host response to the infectious agent.

◆ **Answer 1.3**
An intranuclear inclusion.

◆ **Answer 1.4**
Cytomegalovirus produces large cells with large eosinophilic intranuclear ('owl's eye') inclusion bodies.

◆ **Answer 1.5**
Cytomegalovirus (CMV) is a common infective agent but rarely causes human disease unless a patient is immunocompromised. Symptomatic CMV infection may arise in patients who have not been previously exposed to CMV and then receive a donor kidney from a CMV positive donor at the same time as immunosupressive drug therapy. This patient's immune system needs to be investigated for evidence of immunosupression.

Further investigations show that the patient's T-helper/T-suppressor cell ratio is reduced.

◆ Question 1.6
What further investigations would you now wish to do?

The patient is found to be HIV positive.

◆ Question 1.7
What is a possible mode of transmission in this case?

The patient returns home and is relatively well for 6 months but then develops a febrile illness with breathing difficulties and is admitted under the care of the chest physicians. A bronchoalveolar lavage is performed and a cytological preparation stained by a silver technique has the appearances shown in Figure 1.2.

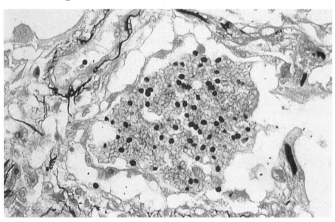

Fig. 1.2

◆ Question 1.8
What infective organism is present now?

◆ Question 1.9
How may this infection be treated?

◆ Question 1.10
What other pathologies may develop in a patient with acquired immunodeficiency syndrome (AIDS)?

Revision

- AIDS, see pp. 219–220

- Cytomegalorivus infection, see pp. 219, 375, 851

- Inflammatory and infective intestinal disorders, see pp. 427–437

◆ Answer 1.6
Serological tests for human immunodeficiency virus (HIV).

◆ Answer 1.7
Intravenous drug abuse. The patient has previously had endocarditis of the tricuspid valve which rarely occurs unless material has been injected into the systemic venous circulation. The other modes of transmission (sexual intercourse and blood products) should also be investigated and the patient should be given appropriate counselling.

◆ Answer 1.8
Pneumocystis carinii.

◆ Answer 1.9
High doses of co-trimoxazole.

◆ Answer 1.10
Many infections can occur such as cerebral toxoplasmosis, atypical mycobacterial infections, systemic fungal infections (such as candida) and parasitic infections of the gastrointestinal tract. Tumours may also occur including lymphoma and Kaposi's sarcoma.

Fits

Six months ago a 22-year-old nurse with no relevant past medical history woke up one morning with a severe headache and found that she had wet the bed during the night. She was so embarrassed that she didn't tell anyone. For the next few months she had further headaches, worse just before her periods.

While on duty she has a 'blackout'. The ward sister is called and recognises immediately that the nurse is having an epileptic fit.

◆ Question 2.1
What features would lead you to recognise an epileptic fit?

The nurse recovers from the fit and is taken back to her room in the nurses' hostel. An urgent appointment is made for her to see the neurologist at the hospital.

◆ Question 2.2
What are the common causes of epilepsy?

The neurologist makes a thorough examination and finds no abnormality. He prescribes phenytoin to control the fits and requests a computerised tomography (CT) scan of the brain. This reveals a 10-mm diameter extrinsic lesion close to and compressing the underlying brain. The density of the lesion is enhanced by contrast medium.

◆ Question 2.3
What is the pathological basis for enhancement of contrast in CT imaging?

The nurse is told that her epilepsy is probably due to a small tumour growing between the brain and the skull. She is told the probable tumour type.

◆ Question 2.4
What is the most likely identity of this tumour?

◆ Answer 2.1
Grand mal epileptic fits are characterised by often violent involuntary repetitive limb movements. The individual loses consciousness and may remain unconscious for some time after the fitting stops. Incontinence is also common.

◆ Answer 2.2
Most cases of epilepsy are idiopathic; this means that there is no identifiable cause. However, each new case must be carefully assessed to determine whether the fits are due to an identifiable local problem warranting specific treatment. Local causes include:

- meningeal scars secondary to previous meningitis
- tumours — primary or metastatic
- old cerebral infarcts.

◆ Answer 2.3
Enhancement of the image by contrast medium indicates a vascularised abnormality, in contrast to a cyst, for example.

◆ Answer 2.4
This is probably a meningioma. Although most are designated benign because they do not invade, compression of the adjacent brain tissue is a serious consequence.

She is referred to the local neurosurgical unit. There the tumour is removed and submitted for histopathological examination (Fig. 2.1).

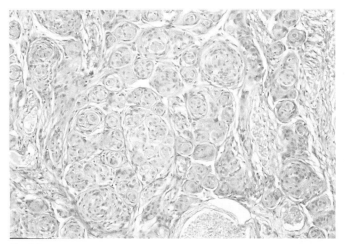

Fig. 2.1

◆ Question 2.5
What type of tumour is it and what is its histogenesis?

The patient made a good postoperative recovery. Anticonvulsant therapy was stopped about 3 months after surgery and, when followed up 6 months later she was free from fits and headaches and had returned to work full-time.

Revision

■ Meningioma, see p. 871

■ Tumour angiogenesis, see pp. 248, 276

◆ Answer 2.5
The histological appearance, characterised by whorls of cells associated with psammoma bodies, is typical of a meningioma. It is derived from the cells of the arachnoid granulations.

Asymptomatic woman

You are the consultant radiologist at a triple assessment clinic in the United Kingdom's National Breast Screening Programme. Over the afternoon you are going to see 10 women who have been called back for further assessment after their initial screening mammogram.

◆ **Question 3.1**
What is triple assessment in breast disease?

Your first patient is a 53-year-old woman, on whom mammography of the left breast has shown the lesion in Figure 3.1.

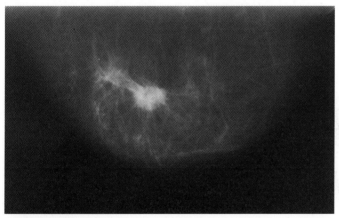

Fig. 3.1

◆ **Question 3.2**
What can you see in Figure 3.1?

◆ **Question 3.3**
Why do cancers show up on mammograms?

Taking a history from the patient, you pick up only that she had a tonsillectomy at 6 years and was treated for a peptic ulcer at age 44. On examination the breasts look normal and contain no masses.

◆ **Question 3.4**
Does this mean that the patient can be reassured and sent home?

You perform stereotactically guided fine-needle aspiration of the lesion (Fig. 3.2).

◆ **Answer 3.1**
It is the correlation of clinical, imaging (mammograms and/or ultrasound) and cytological findings to arrive at a diagnosis.

◆ **Answer 3.2**
It shows a stellate white area, which radiologists recognise as a parenchymal abnormality likely to represent cancer.

◆ **Answer 3.3**
Most of the breast tissue is fatty and is relatively lucent to x-rays. Carcinomas may have radio-opaque calcified areas which show up as white speckles or dense fibrous tissue which causes stellate white areas to be seen.

◆ **Answer 3.4**
No it does not. The point of the scheme is to detect early breast cancer at a stage where it may be impalpable.

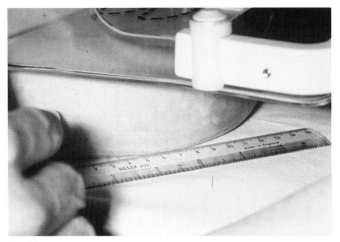

Fig. 3.2

◆ **Question 3.5**
Why do you need stereotactic radiographic guidance of your aspirate?

The fine-needle aspirate is shown in Figure 3.3. The cytopathologist's report reads: 'A highly cellular aspirate consisting of poorly cohesive cells with pleomorphic nuclei, considered diagnostic of malignancy.' You discuss the findings with the patient, who consents to excision biopsy.

◆ **Answer 3.5**
The lesion is impalpable so you would not otherwise know where to direct your needle.

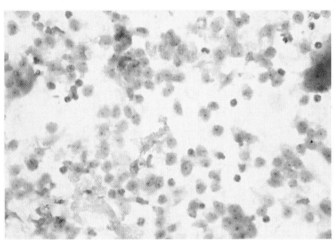

Fig. 3.3

◆ **Question 3.6**
If the lesion is impalpable, how can the surgeon determine what part of the breast tissue to excise?

With her localisation wire taped in place (Fig. 3.4), the patient is taken straight to the operating theatre where the surgeon excises breast tissue under general anaesthesia from around the tip of the guide wire. The specimen is sent immediately to be radiographed, accompanied by the original mammograms.

◆ **Answer 3.6**
A marker biopsy is performed. In this the stereotactic localisation technique is again used, not this time for a fine-needle aspirate, but to insert a hooked wire into this lesion under local anaesthetic.

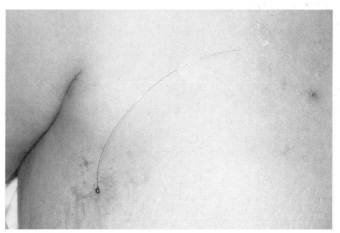

Fig. 3.4

◆ **Question 3.7**
What is the point of radiographing the specimen?

The radiologist reports apparently complete excision to the surgeon in theatre. The patient is woken up and goes home that evening. Two days later, the histopathologist issues the following report:

'This shows a 9-mm maximum diameter grade 1 invasive ductal adenocarcinoma with some microcalcification. No vascular invasion is seen. The tumour extends into the deep resection margin. The surrounding breast tissue shows fibrocystic disease without epithelial proliferation.'

◆ **Question 3.8**
What further procedure does the patient need?

◆ **Question 3.9**
Why does she need the axillary lymph nodes sampling?

The patient opts for wider local excision. This showed a 1-mm diameter area of residual cancer, making her overall tumour diameter 10 mm. The axillary lymph nodes were not involved. The prognosis for a patient with a grade 1 (well-differentiated) tumour of that diameter and stage is excellent, with survival figures similar to patients without breast cancer.

◆ **Answer 3.7**
To make sure that the lesion originally seen in the mammograms has been fully and correctly excised.

◆ **Answer 3.8**
She should be offered completion of the local excision, either by a more extensive local excision or by mastectomy. Patient preference and technical factors will determine which option is taken. In either case she needs to have the axillary lymph nodes sampled on that side.

◆ **Answer 3.9**
Her prognosis can be calculated from the diameter and grade of the primary tumour together with the lymph node status (whether involved by cancer or not). The stage of the tumour can be used to plan adjuvant (hormonal or chemotherapeutic) treatment and radiotherapy.

Revision
- Breast disease, see pp. 523–530
- Breast screening, see pp. 528
- Cytopathology, see pp. 68–70, 527
- Invasion, see pp. 283–284

'My leg gave way'

A mildly obese woman of 75 presents to the Accident and Emergency department with a history of a fall at home. She is a widow who lives alone and she was found by her daughter who visits her daily. The ambulance staff have brought her medication with them, these include medication for hypertension and some analgesics including aspirin and distalgesic.

◆ Question 4.1
What are some common causes of falls in the elderly?

On examination she is alert and lucid, she is in normal cardiac rhythm and her blood pressure is 110/90. She is apyrexial and her palmar creases are pink. She is not jaundiced. Her right leg is shortened and externally rotated and her right hip is painful. She says that as she got out of bed the previous day her leg gave way and she fell to the floor where she remained until found by her daughter about 20 hours later. She has numerous bruises of various ages on legs and arms but no bruising on the hip.

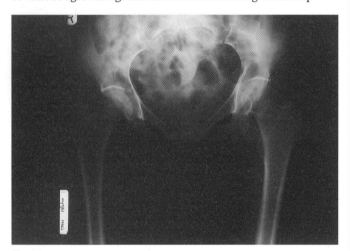

Fig. 4.1

◆ Question 4.2
What is the probable diagnosis? What does the radiograph in Figure 4.1 show?

◆ Question 4.3
What investigations could you perform?

◆ Question 4.4
What is the significance of the pattern of bruising?

She is treated appropriately and is mobilized after 5 days but the next day is found dead in the lavatory.

◆ Answer 4.1
Domestic causes: tripping over furniture, pets, etc.
Confusion: due to drugs, cerebral atrophy, strokes, anaemia, transient ischaemic attacks, hypertension.
Degenerative disease: arthritis, osteoporosis, cardiac dysrhythmias.

◆ Answer 4.2
Shortening and external rotation of a leg with pain in the hip in an elderly patient is generally diagnostic of a fracture of the neck of the femur. This is confirmed in the X-radiograph shown in Figure 4.1. In addition the bone looks 'thinned' (osteopenia).

◆ Answer 4.3
The diagnosis was confirmed with a plain radiograph of the pelvis. Since the condition will require surgery, appropriate tests to ensure that the patient is fit for surgery should be performed, these would include: haemoglobin concentration: urea and electrolytes, chest radiograph. The physical examination should aim to exclude other injuries sustained during the fall as well as the normal full examination.

◆ Answer 4.4
Numerous bruises of different duration are often found in the elderly living alone. Patterns of bruising suggestive of assault should always be considered. The lack of bruising of the hip suggests the possibility that the fracture was spontaneous and the patient may have severe osteoporosis or other bone disease such as carcinoma metastatic to the hip.

◆ **Question 4.5**
What was the treatment?

◆ **Question 4.6**
Is mobilization this soon a good idea?

◆ **Question 4.7**
Should this case be reported to the coroner?

At autopsy she is found to have no systemic disease apart from some granularity of the kidney surfaces, supporting the diagnosis of hypertension.

◆ **Question 4.8**
What major finding do you expect?

◆ **Answer 4.5**
The usual treatment is surgical. This involves total or partial replacement of the hip joint.

◆ **Answer 4.6**
The aim of early mobilization is to prevent further loss of mobility and independence in the patient and particularly to avoid the development of deep vein thrombosis.

◆ **Answer 4.7**
Yes. The death has occurred following an accident and possibly as a result of the accident. Deaths that may be due to an accident must be referred to the coroner, regardless of the time elapsed.

◆ **Answer 4.8**
At autopsy the patient is found to have deep vein thrombosis in the calf of the operated leg, she has a massive pulmonary embolus and severe osteoporosis (Figs 4.2, 4.3, 4.4). Figure 4.2 shows the surgically repaired fracture, Figure 4.3 shows an X-radiograph of the other osteoporotic femur, and Figure 4.4 shows a histological preparation of osteoporotic bone with thin trabeculae.

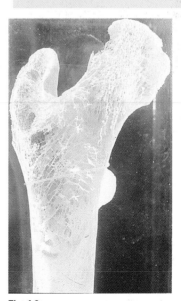

Fig. 4.2   Fig. 4.3

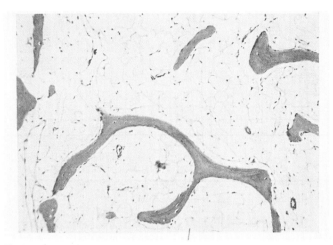

Fig. 4.4

◆ **Question 4.9**
Will the coroner hold an inquest?

Revision

■ Osteoporosis, see pp. 788–789

■ Thrombosis and embolism, see pp. 166–173

■ Autopsy, see pp. 75–76

■ Ageing and death, see pp. 293–304

◆ **Answer 4.9**
The decision to hold an inquest or not is the coroner's prerogative based on the circumstances of the accident, the subsequent clinical history and the post-mortem findings. In this case the pathologist recorded the death as being due to natural causes rather than any severe accident. He felt there was minimum trauma that would not have caused fracture in normal bone and that the whole sequence of events was initiated by her natural disease (osteoporosis). The coroner agreed with this and did not order an inquest.

Pruritus

A 40-year-old woman, married with three healthy children, sees her family doctor because she is finding it difficult to get to sleep at night; her skin itches.

◆ Question 5.1
What conditions are associated with itchy skin (pruritus)?

The patient also complains of episodes of severe pain in the upper abdomen. She is in pain now. The doctor notices that her skin (which is fair), in addition to showing scratch marks, also appears slightly yellow. The sclera of her eyes are also yellow, confirming the suspicion of jaundice. When questioned she comments that her stools are paler than usual.

◆ Question 5.2
What is the significance of pale stools?

A urine sample appears darker than normal, and excess bilirubin is present.

◆ Question 5.3
What is the significance of the excess bilirubin in the urine? How does the presence of bilirubin in the urine assist in the differential diagnosis of jaundice?

The doctor examines the patient's abdomen. There are no masses to feel, but the patient is rather obese. The only abnormality is tenderness in the right hypochondrium. The doctor diagnoses biliary obstruction due to gallstones and makes an urgent appointment for her to be seen by a surgeon.

◆ Question 5.4
Why are gallstones considered to be the most likely cause for the patient's biliary obstruction?

◆ Answer 5.1
Pruritus can be due to skin disorders or systemic illnesses. Skin disorders causing pruritus include allergies, urticaria, and insect bites; in these conditions, the mediator is usually histamine released from mast cells.

◆ Answer 5.2
Pale stools in this clinical context imply that they have a reduced content of stercobilinogen.

◆ Answer 5.3
Bilirubin in the urine is a feature of obstructive jaundice. Pre-hepatic jaundice, for example due to increased formation of bilirubin from haemolysis, does not cause dark urine because the excess bilirubin has not been conjugated in the liver and, therefore, is not sufficiently water soluble to appear in the urine.

◆ Answer 5.4
Gallstones are the commonest cause of biliary obstruction with pain. Viral hepatitis is a common cause of jaundice with dark urine but rarely causes severe pain. Carcinoma of the head of the pancreas, obstructing the common bile duct, is another possibility, but unlikely in the absence of weight loss.

The surgeon arranges for an ultrasound examination of the abdomen (Fig. 5.1).

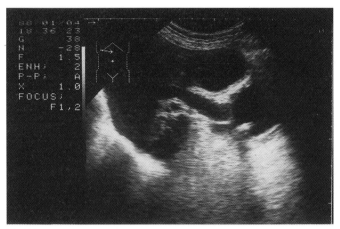

Fig. 5.1

◆ **Question 5.5**
What abnormality is present?

The patient has a cholecystectomy with removal of the stone lodged in the bile duct. She makes an uneventful recovery. Her jaundice clears, but she is still intermittently troubled by pruritus.

Five years later, the patient attends her doctor's clinic. She feels tired, partly because the pruritus has become intolerable. Her doctor notices that the patient is jaundiced.

◆ **Question 5.6**
Could the patient have developed further gallstones?

The doctor finds, on examination, yellow nodules up to 2 mm in diameter on the patient's upper eyelids. The doctor takes a blood sample and sends it to the local hospital laboratory for tests of liver biochemistry and for measurement of the serum cholesterol. The results are:

	Patient's values	Normal range
Alanine aminotransferase (ALT)	55 U/l	5–40 U/l
Alkaline phosphatase	630 U/l	30–110 U/l
Bilirubin	28 μmol/l	5–17 μmol/l
Albumin	39 g/l	35–50 g/l
Cholesterol	7 mmol/l	<c.6.5 mmol/l

◆ **Question 5.7**
How should you interpret these findings?

◆ **Answer 5.5**
There is a gallstone obstructing the common bile duct, with dilatation of the duct proximally.

◆ **Answer 5.6**
Yes, but it is unlikely. Gallstones rarely develop after cholecystectomy, but they can form in the bile ducts.

◆ **Answer 5.7**
The serum cholesterol is high. (The doctor suspected that the nodules around the eyes were xanthelasma — nodules of fat-laden macrophages — indicative of hyperlipidaemia.) The liver biochemistry suggests biliary obstruction rather than hepatitis; the alkaline phosphatase is disproportionately high compared with the transaminases.

The doctor refers the patient to the local hepatologist. The hepatologist performs further investigations. The results are: autoantibody screen — anti-smooth muscle antibody negative, anti-nuclear antibody negative, anti-mitochondrial antibody positive; serum immunoglobulins — IgG normal, IgM elevated; hepatitis virus screen — IgG hepatitis A virus antibody positive, all markers for hepatitis viruses B and C negative.

◆ **Question 5.8**
What is the most likely diagnosis?

Having checked that the prothrombin time is within normal limits, the hepatologist performs a liver biopsy (Fig. 5.2).

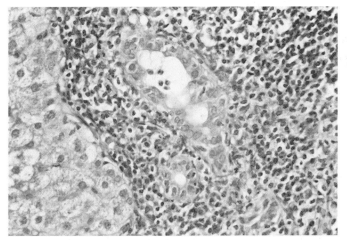

Fig. 5.2

◆ **Question 5.9**
Do the histological features support a diagnosis of primary biliary cirrhosis?

The diagnosis is explained to the patient. She asks if the disease could have been caused by her previous gallstone problem.

◆ **Answer 5.8**
The most likely diagnosis is primary biliary cirrhosis. The features supporting this diagnosis are the anti-mitochondrial antibody (present in c.95% of cases) and the elevated IgM, coupled with the previous serum biochemistry results.

◆ **Answer 5.9**
First, it is not essential for the liver to be cirrhotic; this is a late complication of the disease. The destruction of small bile ducts by lymphocytes is virtually diagnostic of primary biliary cirrhosis. This histological reaction reflects the autoimmune process in which biliary epithelium is the target. Other features appearing as the disease evolves are granulomas, ductular proliferation and fibrosis, and eventually cirrhosis.

◆ **Question 5.10**

What is the relationship between gallstones and primary biliary cirrhosis?

The patient is prescribed penicillamine.

◆ **Question 5.11**

What is the rationale for using penicillamine in primary biliary cirrhosis?

The patient still suffers from itching.

◆ **Question 5.12**

What is the cause of this patient's pruritus?

Revision

■ Jaundice, see pp. 456–457

■ Gallstones, see pp. 477–479

■ Primary biliary cirrhosis, see p. 468

■ Autoimmune diseases, see pp. 204–208

◆ **Answer 5.10**

There is no direct relationship. Gallstones and primary biliary cirrhosis are more common in females, but the conditions are not related.

◆ **Answer 5.11**

Penicillamine interferes with collagen synthesis and will, therefore, theoretically delay the onset of cirrhosis. There is also evidence that penicillamine will ameliorate the inflammatory process. Finally, penicillamine is a chelating agent and will remove from the liver potentially hepatotoxic copper which accumulates as a result of biliary obstruction.

◆ **Answer 5.12**

Pruritus is a well-known manifestation of cholestatic liver diseases. It is often present without clinically evident jaundice and is probably due to accumulation in the skin of a biliary constituent other than bilirubin, such as bile salts.

Failure to thrive

It is February and the second male child of a couple is 3 months old. The pregnancy and birth were normal. The health visitor and parents are concerned, however, because the baby's weight gain is slow and he has a 'chesty' cough. His temperature is 36.7°C. The health visitor advises the parents to take the baby to see their general practitioner.

◆ **Question 6.1**
What is the diagnostic significance of the presenting features?

The GP examines the baby. The weight is 3.9 kg. The lungs are resonant to percussion, but coarse crackles are heard. The general practitioner notices that the mother's fingers are tar-stained and asks if she smokes: she does. The mother is told that cigarette smoke is not only bad for her but also for her baby and that this is probably the cause of her baby's cough. Nevertheless, amoxycillin is prescribed and the mother is told to bring the baby back if her baby's cough doesn't clear up and his weight doesn't increase.

Two weeks later the mother returns. The baby's cough is worse and his weight is falling. The GP arranges an urgent appointment in the paediatric clinic of the local hospital.

◆ **Question 6.2**
What are the most likely diagnoses, assuming that there are no other significant findings?

◆ **Question 6.3**
What is the commonest congenital disorder causing pulmonary and gastrointestinal problems?

The paediatrician arranges for a chest radiograph and for a 'sweat test'.

◆ **Question 6.4**
What is the rationale for these investigations?

The chest X-ray shows no abnormality. The 'sweat test' shows that the sweat sodium concentration is 105 mmol/l (it is usually greater than 70 mmol/l in cystic fibrosis). The paediatrician tells the parents that the baby has cystic fibrosis and that he will require treatment indefinitely. The parents are very upset, and ask about the cause of the disease.

◆ **Question 6.5**
What is the cause of cystic fibrosis?

◆ **Answer 6.1**
Failure to thrive is a common feature of many disorders affecting infants. It is potentially serious and the underlying cause needs identification. Many infants, and adults, develop respiratory infections in winter; in spite of the baby's normal temperature, the cough may be due to a respiratory tract infection and it may require treatment.

◆ **Answer 6.2**
Although the respiratory symptoms and the failure to thrive may be unrelated, it is possible that the child has a condition affecting both the gut and the lungs. Also, in young children, the possibility must be considered that the illness may be due in whole or in part to some congenital defect.

◆ **Answer 6.3**
Cystic fibrosis (mucoviscidosis).

◆ **Answer 6.4**
The chest radiograph is necessary to detect lung abnormalities such as pneumonic consolidation. The 'sweat test', a measurement of the sodium concentration in sweat, is a good screening test for cystic fibrosis.

◆ **Answer 6.5**
Cystic fibrosis is, in Caucasians, the commonest serious genetic disease (prevalence approximately 1:2500). It is due to a mutation in the cystic fibrosis transmembrane conductance regulator gene on the long arm of chromosome 7. This leads to impaired chloride ion and water transport across the membranes of epithelial cells. This results in abnormally viscous exocrine secretions. Involvement of the pancreas impairs digestion and, therefore, is responsible for failure to thrive in infancy. The viscous bronchial secretions block airways and promote infections.

The parents ask if their other son, who is 3 years old, will be affected. He seems quite well at the moment. They also wonder about the risk in further pregnancies.

◆ Question 6.6
What is the mode of inheritance and what is the risk in future pregnancies?

The parents ask about treatment for their baby. The paediatrician explains that physiotherapy and antibiotics will be necessary to help get rid of the chest infection, and that the treatment will be required to restore acceptable weight gain.

◆ Question 6.7
What can be done to improve the baby's gain?

The baby's condition improves. To reduce the risk of serious chest infections he has measles and influenza A immunisation, and continues with regular physiotherapy. Despite these measures, he has several serious respiratory tract infections during the next 5 years, requiring admission to hospital on three occasions.

◆ Question 6.8
What are the long-term pulmonary complications of cystic fibrosis?

◆ Question 6.9
What is the pathogenesis of these changes?

◆ Question 6.10
If the baby survives into adulthood, which is very likely with modern therapy, what would you consider to be the most likely explanation for finding, at that time, significant proteinuria on routine urine testing?

Revision

- Cystic fibrosis, see pp. 139–141
- Inheritance of genetic disorders, see p. 45
- Bronchiectasis, see p. 388
- Amyloid, see pp. 159–162

◆ Answer 6.6
Cystic fibrosis is an autosomal recessive disorder. Both copies of the gene must be defective for the disease to occur. The parents should be told that:

- their apparently healthy 3-year-old son is probably unaffected, but the disease may appear in older children and young adults; he should probably have a 'sweat test'
- the risk is 1:4 pregnancies; it cannot be assumed that, because they have one affected child, the other 3 would be unaffected
- future pregnancies can be screened for cystic fibrosis by DNA analysis of chorionic villous biopsies and the parents counselled when the result is known.

◆ Answer 6.7
He needs replacement therapy to compensate for the impaired pancreatic exocrine secretions. This is available as enteric-coated pancreatic extracts. This will improve his digestion and, hence, intestinal absorption.

◆ Answer 6.8
The principal dangers are the development of bronchiectasis and pulmonary hypertension.

◆ Answer 6.9
Bronchiectasis is due to inflammatory weakening of the bronchial wall, with destruction of elastic tissue and smooth muscle, leading to persistent dilatation with necrotising infection. Pulmonary hypertension results from a combination of increased pulmonary vascular resistance due to pulmonary fibrosis and increased bronchopulmonary vascular shunting.

◆ Answer 6.10
Amyloid deposition of AA type. This is a well-recognised complication of chronic inflammatory conditions such as bronchiectasis.

New fever on old

A 77-year-old man is admitted to hospital after a home visit by his general practitioner. When interviewed he is confused and unable to give a coherent history. His wife says that he has been unwell for 3 weeks during which time he has been feverish and lethargic. He had worked as a clerk in the local council housing department until his retirement aged 65 years. As a child he had had rheumatic fever but had had no major illnesses since then. He had smoked cigarettes as a youth but had given up during the Second World War.

On examination the patient has a temperature of 38.2°. He has an apex beat which is displaced laterally and a faint ejection systolic murmur. Crackles are heard at the bases of both lungs. The abdomen and nervous system are unremarkable.

◆ Question 7.1
What investigations would you order?

The patient did not produce any sputum for culture. The urine is sterile but a microscopic haematuria was noted. Culture of blood at 24 hours was negative but further culture is being carried out. The patient's temperature chart is shown in Figure 7.1.

The patient has become semiconscious, his heart rate has increased and his urine output has fallen.

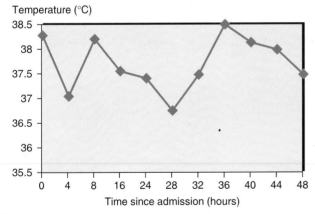

Temperature (°C)

Time since admission (hours)

Fig. 7.1

◆ Question 7.2
What treatment would you now consider?

◆ Answer 7.1
This patient has a fever with no obvious focus of infection so investigations should be directed towards finding that source. Samples of urine, blood and sputum (if present) should be sent for culture. A chest radiograph should be performed. A temperature chart should be kept as the pattern of fever can sometimes give clues as to the aetiology.

◆ Answer 7.2
Although no focus of infection has been found yet the patient's condition is getting worse. Specimens have been sent for culture so blind broad-spectrum antibiotic therapy could be started.

The patient's condition continues to deteriorate and he dies. An autopsy is performed at the request of the local coroner because the doctors who cared for the patient cannot give a cause of death. Figure 7.2 shows the lesion to the spleen discovered at autopsy.

Figure 7.3 shows a lesion present in one of the kidneys.

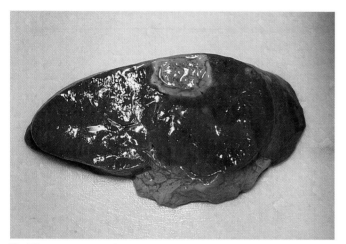

Fig. 7.2

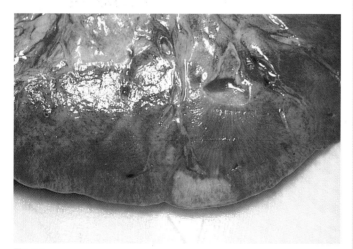

Fig. 7.3

◆ **Question 7.3**
What pathological process could cause lesions with this distribution and shape?

◆ **Answer 7.3**
The lesions in both organs are at the periphery and both organs have an end artery blood supply; the lesion in the kidney has a definite 'wedge' shape. These features suggest that the lesions are infarcts. The infarcts could be caused by thrombosis in the vessels or by emboli; since more than one organ is affected embolization is the most probable process.

The appearances of the aortic valve are shown in Figure 7.4.

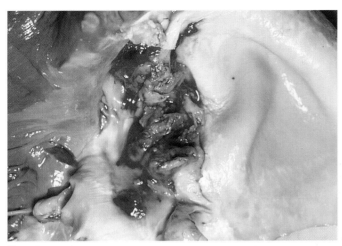

Fig. 7.4

◆ **Question 7.4**
What lesions are present?

◆ **Question 7.5**
What is the likely cause of this patient's fever?

◆ **Question 7.6**
What is the likely cause of the pathology in the spleen and kidney?

◆ **Question 7.7**
What further investigations does the pathologist need to carry out?

Histology of the valve vegetations show Gram-positive cocci and culture produces a growth of *Staphylococcus aureus*.

◆ **Question 7.8**
What other organisms may cause infective endocarditis?

◆ **Question 7.9**
What past illness may have predisposed this patient to developing infective endocarditis?

◆ **Question 7.10**
What other physical signs, not mentioned in this case, may be present in infective endocarditis?

◆ **Answer 7.4**
There are vegetations on the valve cusps.

◆ **Answer 7.5**
Infective endocarditis.

◆ **Answer 7.6**
Emboli from the valve vegetations.

◆ **Answer 7.7**
Samples of the vegetations should be sent for culture and examined histologically.

◆ **Answer 7.8**
Many sorts of organisms can cause infective endocarditis in special circumstances, such as immunocompromised hosts and intravenous drug users, but the commoner organisms are *Staph. aureus, Streptococcus faecalis, Strep. mitior, Strep. mutans, Strep. sanguis, Candida albicans* and *Coxiella burnettii*.

◆ **Answer 7.9**
Rheumatic fever producing scarring of the aortic valve.

◆ **Answer 7.10**
Splinter haemorrhages in the fingernails and digital clubbing.

Revision

- Rheumatic valvulitis, see pp. 341, 814–815
- Infective endocarditis, see pp. 344–350
- Embolism and infarction, see pp. 169–178
- Autopsy, see pp. 75–76

Weight gain

A 49-year-old man presents with a 1-year history of weight gain, about which he says he is miserable. He has tried several diets but has gained 15 kg over the last year. He does not think that he is eating excessively; for one thing, his mouth is too sore.

On examination, his general build is as shown in Figure 8.1.

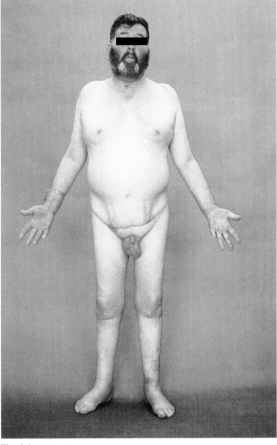

Fig. 8.1

◆ **Question 8.1**
What abnormality can you see?

◆ **Answer 8.1**
He has a truncal distribution of fat while his legs are thin.

His thighs show the abnormality in Figure 8.2.

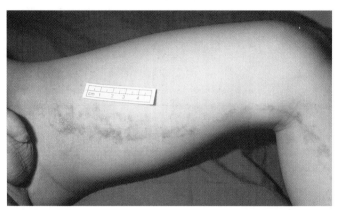

Fig. 8.2

◆ **Question 8.2**
What abnormality can you see?

You look in his mouth and see the lesion shown in Figure 8.3.

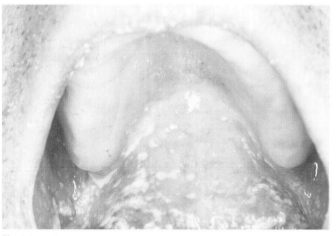

Fig. 8.3

◆ **Question 8.3**
What is this?

You take scraping from the mouth and send them for microscopy and culture.

◆ **Question 8.4**
How do you tie these abnormal findings together?

You arrange for urinary analysis including 17-hydroxysteroid estimation, blood biochemistry including cortisol and adrenocortico-trophic hormone (ACTH) levels. The results show moderate hyperglycaemia, mild glycosuria, massively elevated blood cortisol and urinary 17-hydroxysteroids, and depressed blood ACTH.

◆ **Answer 8.2**
The purple/white stripes down the medial surface of the thighs are lichen striatus.

◆ **Answer 8.3**
In this edentulous mouth there are white deposits on the hard pallet and gums. They are probably oral 'thrush' which is infection by Candida, a yeast.

◆ **Answer 8.4**
When a patient has multiple abnormalities, you should always consider first whether a single problem could explain them all. In this case, the truncal obesity, weight gain, depression, striae and oral candidiasis are all potentially related to elevated blood glucocorticoids (Cushing's syndrome or disease).

◆ **Question 8.5**
What do these results indicate?

After CT scan of the retroperitoneum showed a mass in the left adrenal the patient underwent an adrenalectomy on that side. The excised adrenal gland is shown in Figure 8.4.

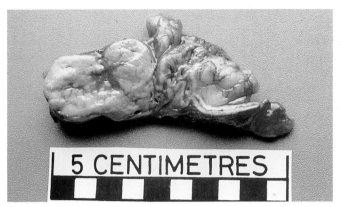

5 CENTIMETRES

Fig. 8.4

◆ **Question 8.6**
What does this show?

The histopathology report states that an adrenal cortical neoplasm was found, with no specific histological features to suggest malignancy.

◆ **Question 8.7**
In a patient with an adrenal cortical neoplasm what general features would suggest malignancy of the neoplasm?

The patient made a complete recovery.

◆ **Question 8.8**
What is the importance of suspecting and detecting adrenal cortical neoplasms?

Revision

■ Cushing's syndrome, see pp. 497–499

■ Adrenal cortex tumours, see p. 499

◆ **Answer 8.5**
The elevated blood cortisol and urinary 17-hydroxysteroids indicate, in the absence of exogenous steroid administration, that the patient has either Cushing's disease or syndrome. Cushing's *disease* is due to the pituitary producing excess ACTH. The patient's depressed ACTH rules out this condition. The patient therefore has Cushing's disease due to an adrenal problem.

◆ **Answer 8.6**
It shows a yellow coloured nodule in the adrenal cortex typical of an adrenal cortical neoplasm.

◆ **Answer 8.7**   Different
Excess production of androgens or oestrogens, large tumour size and metastasis at the time of surgery all point to malignancy.

◆ **Answer 8.8**
They may, by secreting steroids, give rise to uncontrollable hypertension, a diabetic state (as in this patient), immunosuppression, psychiatric disturbances and osteoporosis. Hypertension is the main problem caused by neoplasms which secrete aldosterone (Conn's syndrome), while the immunosuppressive and diabetogenic effects are more marked with ones which secrete glucocorticoids, as in this case.

Itchy nipple

A 37-year-old woman presents to your surgical outpatient clinic with a 3-week history of an itchy red nipple on the left (Fig. 9.1). She has a past history of eczema as a child, and of appendicectomy. She is married with no children.

◆ **Question 9.1**
What is the differential diagnosis of nipples that look like Figure 9.1?

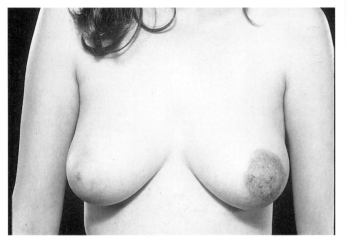

Fig. 9.1

You conduct a thorough examination of the patient. The breast contains no masses and the axillary lymph nodes are not enlarged. There are no other significant findings.

◆ **Question 9.2**
What investigations should you do next?

◆ **Answer 9.1**
Paget's disease of the nipple must always be excluded; true eczema can occur at the nipple but this is a rare site and when it occurs it is commonly bilateral. In older women there is a very rare condition called erosive adenoma of the nipple to consider also.

◆ **Answer 9.2**
You need to take a good biopsy of the nipple under local anaesthetic and should order mammograms. There is no point in performing fine-needle aspiration because you cannot feel any lesion to aspirate.

The mammograms are reported as being rather dense and difficult to interpret due to the patient's relatively young age. The left breast, however, contains linear tracks of coarse calcification consistent with intraduct carcinoma in all four quadrants.

The histological appearance of the nipple biopsy is shown in Figure 9.2.

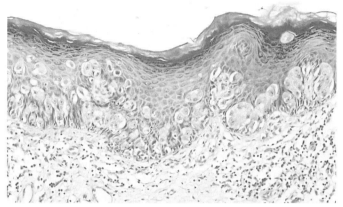

Fig. 9.2

◆ **Question 9.3**
What does this show?

Special stains show the abnormal cells in the skin of the nipple to contain mucin.

◆ **Question 9.4**
What is the significance of these cells?

The surgeon recommends that the patient should undergo left simple mastectomy.

◆ **Question 9.5**
Why does the patient need a mastectomy for a lesion that may not even be invasive?

◆ **Answer 9.3**
It shows infiltration of the epidermis by large cells with pale cytoplasm and pleomorphic nuclei.

◆ **Answer 9.4**
They signify Paget's disease of the nipple, a condition where malignant adenocarcinoma cells grow up the breast ducts and lactiferous sinuses to infiltrate the nipple. The underlying lesion in the breast is intraduct carcinoma with or without an invasive component.

◆ **Answer 9.5**
Multiquadrant disease has been documented in this patient, making local excision impossible. She is not suitable for subcutaneous mastectomy because the skin of the nipple is involved by malignant cells.

A simple mastectomy is performed, which confirms histologically the diagnosis of Paget's disease of the nipple and shows appearances like that seen in Figure 9.3 in all four quadrants.

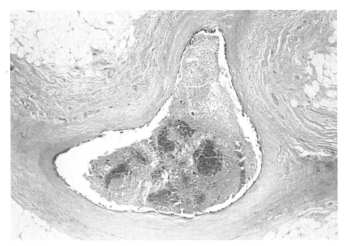

Fig. 9.3

◆ Question 9.6
What does Figure 9.3 show?

Apart from the ductal carcinoma-in-situ the mastectomy specimen shows no invasive carcinoma.

◆ Question 9.7
What is the prognosis for this patient?

◆ Question 9.8
What advice should she be given?

Revision

- Paget's disease of the nipple, see p. 546
- Ductal carcinoma-in-situ, see pp. 540–541
- In-situ neoplasia, see p. 254
- Dystrophic calcification, see p. 235

◆ Answer 9.6
It shows a duct filled by large malignant cells with extensive central necrosis. This is the appearance of ductal carcinoma-in-situ of the comedo necrosis type.

◆ Answer 9.7
The mastectomy should be curative since she had only in-situ disease without invasion.

◆ Answer 9.8
The intraduct carcinoma in the left breast is a marker of increased risk for the subsequent development of carcinoma in the remaining breast, indicating approximately a four-fold increased risk compared with normal women. Breast self-examination and mammograms can increase the chance of detecting any neoplasm at an early stage.

'Might it be due to my job?'

A local general practitioner has referred a 45-year-old man with a 3-week history of haematuria to the consultant urologist. The patient's full blood count result sent (thoughtfully) in advance to the clinic shows hypochromic microcytic anaemia.

◆ Question 10.1
On its own, what does that imply?

Further history from the patient indicates that he has been healthy until the present episode of red coloured urine. He smokes about 20 cigarettes per day and has worked all his life as a coking plant labourer for the National Coal Board. Symptomatic enquiry yields no additional symptoms and physical examination is normal apart from slight pallor of the mucous membranes.

◆ Question 10.2
What would be appropriate investigations to request?

The urine proves to be sterile, but the cytopathologist reports the presence of malignant cells in the urine. Further tests include an intravenous urogram, which is a contrast radiograph of the kidneys, ureters and bladder. This is reported as showing a possible filling defect in the left renal pelvis.

◆ Question 10.3
Where might the malignant cells come from? How can their source be determined?

On cystoscopy, the bladder appears normal and random biopsies are taken. After cannulation of the ureters the patient is transferred to the radiographic department where the retrograde pyelogram (which consists of injecting contrast medium up the ureters) shows up a papillary growth in the left renal pelvis only. Two days later the histopathologist reports on the bladder biopsies as showing normal urothelium.

◆ Question 10.4
Taken together, what do these findings imply?

The patient undergoes a left nephroureterectomy. At the weekly histopathology conference, the histopathologist demonstrates the patient's sections. The renal pelvis is shown in Figure 10.1.

◆ Answer 10.1
It suggests that, excepting rarities, the cause is likely to be iron deficiency, which may result through blood loss.

◆ Answer 10.2
Microscopy and culture of the urine in the microbiology laboratory (to check whether the haematuria is due to infection) and cytological examination of the urine (to check for malignant cells) should be arranged.

◆ Answer 10.3
They are likely to be from the transitional epithelium which lines the ureters, bladder and urethra. Of these, the bladder is the commonest source; the patient should be admitted for a cystoscopy. He should also have a retrograde pyelogram to check out the left renal pelvis.

◆ Answer 10.4
They point strongly to carcinoma of the renal pelvis.

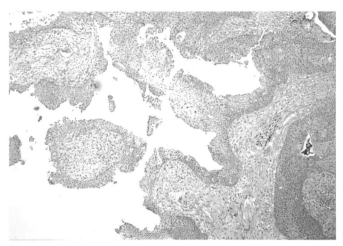

Fig. 10.1

◆ **Question 10.5**
What does this show?

The patient says he has heard from his trades union representative that his occupation can cause cancer.

◆ **Question 10.6**
What advice should be given? What are the known causes of transitional cell carcinoma?

After an uneventful recovery, the patient re-presents 2 years later with frequency of micturition, haematuria and weight loss. At cystoscopy, the lesion in Figure 10.2 is seen.

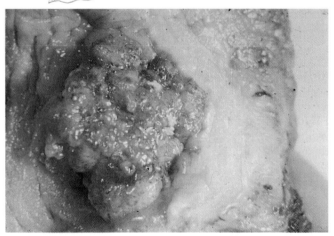

Fig. 10.2

◆ **Question 10.7**
What is it?

Bimanual palpation of the tumour both before and after fulguration (diathermy excision/biopsy for histology), reveals there is residual tumour, fixed to the muscle of the bladder wall.

◆ **Answer 10.5**
It shows a papillary transitional cell carcinoma. There is no invasion of the lamina propria and the tumour is well differentiated, so the prognosis is favourable.

◆ **Answer 10.6**
Occupational exposure to tars and other hydrocarbons encountered in the coal products industry is a known cause of transitional cell carcinoma as is tar from cigarette smoking. Compounds used in the dye industry can also be responsible. He may be entitled to compensation.

◆ **Answer 10.7**
It is a papillary carcinoma, almost certainly of transitional cell type.

◆ Question 10.8
What does this imply about the stage of the tumour?

The histopathology report confirms this impression, showing moderately differentiated transitional cell carcinoma invading into deep muscle. The clinical staging of bladder cancer generally shows good correlation with the histological stage due to the accuracy of bimanual palpation in its assessment. Postoperatively the patient develops lymphoedema of his left leg, shown on CT scanning to be due to massive lymph node metastases (Fig. 10.3) in the left common iliac chain compressing the pelvic veins. His condition deteriorates rapidly and he dies.

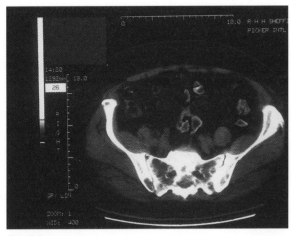

Fig. 10.3

The new house officer issues a death certificate as shown below:
1a Carcinomatosis
1b Transitional cell carcinoma of the bladder
1c Industrial exposure to hydrocarbons

◆ Question 10.9
What is wrong with this?

Revision

- Cytopathy, see pp. 68–70

- Transitional cell carcinoma of bladder, see pp. 654–655

- Chemical carcinogens, see pp. 266–268

- Tumour staging, see pp. 65, 289–290

- Invasion, see pp. 283–284

◆ Answer 10.8
It implies that there is invasion of deep bladder-wall muscle.

◆ Answer 10.9
The house officer should have reported the case to the coroner, who investigates all deaths which may be due to industrial injury (including chemical exposure). The coroner would arrange for a post-mortem to be performed and conduct an inquest into the death.

Feeling the cold

You are the general practitioner for a 64-year-old lady. The patient has been receiving injections of vitamin B12 from your district nurse for the last 8 years.

◆ Question 11.1
What are these for?

The nurse telephones you to say that she is worried about the patient. She is complaining of feeling the cold and appears to have lost interest in looking after her house properly. You visit the patient at home: it is in a mess compared with the last time you visited. The patient (Fig. 11.1) complains that the housework is too much for her and that she never seems to get round to it. Her voice is croaky.

◆ Answer 11.1
They are to replace dietary vitamin B12 which has failed to be absorbed, virtually always as a result of the atrophic gastritis which causes pernicious anaemia.

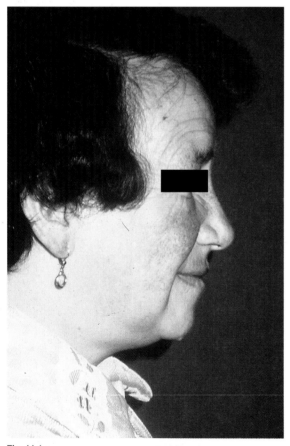

Fig. 11.1

◆ **Question 11.2**
Taking into account these observations and Figure 11.1, what is the most likely diagnosis?

On examination you note that her pulse is 60, she has swollen ankles and her skin is very faintly yellow.

◆ **Question 11.3**
Do these features fit with the diagnosis?

You examine the neck and find the thyroid to be impalpable. You explain to the patient that you are going to send off some blood tests which may well reveal the cause of her symptoms.

◆ **Question 11.4**
What are the most appropriate tests to do?

The results show an elevated TSH level, slightly depressed T_4 and the presence of auto-antibodies to thyroglobulin and thyroid microsomal components.

◆ **Question 11.5**
What does elevation of the TSH imply and what is the diagnosis?

You visit the patient and explain that she will need to take thyroid replacement in the form of oral thyroxine, on a permanent basis.

◆ **Question 11.6**
What are the special considerations when prescribing thyroxine to an elderly patient?

You visit the patient in 1 month's time to see how she is and check her blood T_4 and TSH levels. She has started getting about more, her face is a lot less puffy and she is more talkative. Her granddaughter who is a medical student has told her that her hypothyroidism could be related to her pernicious anaemia.

◆ **Question 11.7**
Is she right?

◆ **Answer 11.2**
A diagnosis of hypothyroidism could explain her puffy face, dry hair, loss of lateral eyebrow hair, lethargy, depression, croaky voice and feeling the cold.

◆ **Answer 11.3**
Yes they do. Hypothyroidism can lead to bradycardia and heart failure. Slow metabolism can lead to carotinaemia giving rise to a yellow colour which is not jaundice.

◆ **Answer 11.4**
The patient in any case needs her full blood count, vitamin B12 and folate levels doing because she has pernicious anaemia. Her blood biochemistry should be checked since she is slightly yellow coloured. The best test to reveal most cases of hypothyroidism is radioimmunoassay for thyroid stimulating hormone (TSH) levels. Her blood T_4 level and thyroid auto-antibodies should also be checked.

◆ **Answer 11.5**
An elevated TSH indicates that thyroid secretion is deficient and that the pituitary is trying to compensate by secreting more TSH to stimulate the gland. The thyroid auto-antibodies indicate that the patient has Hashimoto's thyroiditis.

◆ **Answer 11.6**
The dose has to be cautiously low. If hyperthyroidism were caused by relative overdosage, this could precipitate cardiac dysrhythmias, myocardial ischaemia and heart failure.

◆ **Answer 11.7**
Yes she is. Both are organ-specific autoimmune diseases which occur predominantly in females and are associated with certain HLA types, including HLA-B8 and -DR5. Patients with one organ-specific autoimmune disease are at increased risk of developing other ones.

The patient makes a good recovery on thyroxine replacement. Even her swollen ankles return to normal.

◆ Question 11.8
What does this indicate about the cause of her previous congestive cardiac failure?

◆ Question 11.9
In a patient with Hashimoto's thyroiditis what other diseases are found with increased frequency?

◆ Answer 11.8
It indicates that the hypothyroidism was causing this.

◆ Answer 11.9
We have already mentioned one organ-specific autoimmune disease. Others include type 2 diabetes mellitus, vitiligo (patches of skin depigmentation) (Fig. 11.2), alopecia areata (patchy hair loss) and Addison's disease (adrenal failure). There is also an increased risk of thyroid lymphoma.

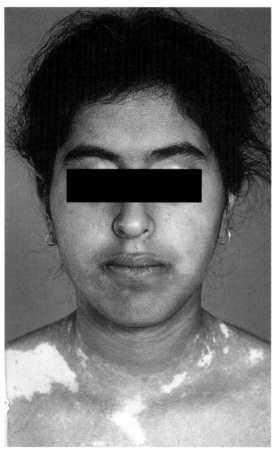

Fig. 11.2

Revision

- Autoimmune disease, see pp. 204–208

- Megaloblastic anaemia, see pp. 703–705, 706–707

- Hashimoto's thyroiditis, see pp. 506–507

- HLA haplotypes and disease, see pp. 31–35, 143

Testicular swelling

An 18-year-old man presents in the Accident and Emergency department with a painful, swollen right testicle. He gives no history of trauma and says that it began with discomfort whilst cycling and is now very painful and tender. On examination there is mild scrotal swelling and the testis is very tender, swollen and retracted.

◆ Question 12.1
What is the differential diagnosis?

He is admitted under the surgeons who explore the scrotum and resect the testis shown in Figure 12.1.

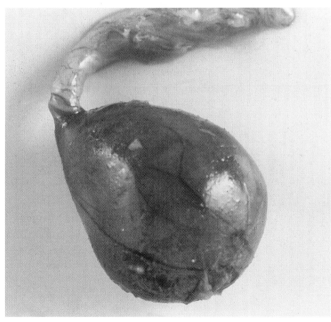

Fig. 12.1

◆ Question 12.2
What alternatives are there to surgical resection?

◆ Question 12.3
What is the pathogenesis of this condition?

◆ Answer 12.1
The differential diagnosis of swellings in the testis include:

- hydrocoele; but this should not be painful and should occur in older patients
- haematoma; but this should have a history of trauma
- tumours; should not be an acute history and generally not painful
- torsion; this is a classical history for torsion, but the other possibilities should not be forgotten.

◆ Answer 12.2
Sometimes it is possible to feel the twist in the spermatic cord and to uncoil this. The main difficulty is that it is very painful if you get it wrong. There is, however, some point in attempting correction since the viability of the testis is at stake.

◆ Answer 12.3
In torsion the testis rotates on the spermatic cord and this compresses the lowest pressure vascular system which is the lymphatics and veins. These, of course, are the return vessels and if these are occluded the arteries will continue to pass blood into the organ causing it to swell. Oedema eventually restricts the arterial supply, causing further pain due to ischaemia. The organ now has a very short time before anoxia causes tissue death. This time is variable but the sooner the situation is corrected the more likely it is that the testis will remain viable and will not need resection. Torsion is often due to excess mobility of the testis and it is advisable to fix the testis, (and the one on the other side), to the wall of the scrotum to prevent similar events in the future.

◆ **Question 12.4**

What is the pathology and treatment of testicular tumours?

◆ **Question 12.5**

Is there a comparable range of pathology in the ovary?

Age

Revision

■ Ischaemia, see pp. 114, 163–173

■ Infarction, see pp. 173–178

■ Testicular tumours, see pp. 605–613

■ Torsion, see p. 176

◆ **Answer 12.4**

Testicular tumours always require resection. Teratomas are the most common in boys of this age, seminomas are more common in the third and fourth decades and lymphomas are the most likely diagnosis in the sixth decade onwards. There are numerous other tumours, but these, and mixtures and variants of them, are the most common. Their classification is complex and depends on grading using both histological features and degree of differentiation. Their prognosis and treatment depends both on grade and stage at presentation. A particular predisposing factor for testicular tumours, at least seminomas and teratomas, is maldescent; even when this has been corrected surgically the testis (and the *contralateral* testis) is still at risk of tumour development subsequently. Remember that lymph drainage of the scrotum is to the inguinal nodes while lymph drainage of the testis is to the para-aortic nodes, so even advanced testicular cancer may present without obvious nodal involvement externally.

◆ **Answer 12.5**

The ovary produces a similar range of tumours but the commonest are epithelial tumours that are usually cystic. These include the serous and mucinous cystic tumours that range from cystic adenomas to adenocarcinomas. Teratomas in the ovary are more often well differentiated than those in the testis and may produce quite complex structures filled with skin, hair and teeth called dermoid cysts. Torsion may also occur in the ovary, particularly if there is a tumour. This may then present clinically as an acute abdomen.

A sudden death

A 54-year-old taxi driver falls to the ground in a shopping mall. Shop staff, trained in first aid, attend and commence cardiopulmonary resuscitation because they cannot detect any pulse or respiratory effort. An ambulance arrives within 10 minutes and the subject is transported to the nearest hospital whilst ambulance staff continue the resuscitative efforts. On arrival in the Accident and Emergency department he is making no respiratory effort and is in asystole. Full resuscitative measures are implemented but there is no response and he is declared dead. His wife, who was with him at the time of the collapse, says that he had not seen a doctor for at least 2 years and appeared to be well before his collapse. He had smoked 20 cigarettes a day for most of his adult life.

◆ **Question 13.1**
What are the common causes of sudden non-traumatic death?

The senior house officer phones the patient's GP to inform him of the death and allow him to make appropriate support resources available to the patient's widow.

◆ **Question 13.2**
Under the medicolegal system of England and Wales will the GP be able to give a medical certificate of the cause of death?

The SHO refers the case to the local coroner who asks a pathologist to perform an autopsy examination.

◆ **Question 13.3**
What training do pathologists have?

Fig. 13.1 shows the appearance of the opened left ventricle at autopsy. The mitral valve in closer view is shown in Fig. 13.2.

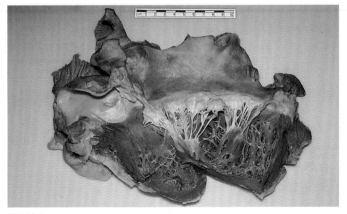

Fig. 13.1

◆ **Answer 13.1**
Cardiac arrhythmias due to ischaemic heart disease, ruptured aortic aneurysm, subarachnoid haemorrhage.

◆ **Answer 13.2**
No. Doctors may only give a certificate of the cause of death if they have seen the deceased in the 14 days before their death and if they consider that they know the cause of death. Neither of these criteria are fulfilled in this case. Since the deceased had not seen his doctor for at least 2 years it is unlikely that the GP could give a cause of death in any medicolegal system.

◆ **Answer 13.3**
Pathologists train as doctors and practise clinical medicine for at least a year after qualification. They then undergo specialist training in pathology which in Britain lasts at least 5 years and involves passing examinations to become a Member of the Royal College of Pathologists.

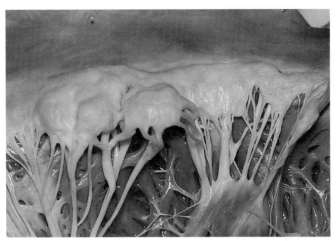

Fig. 13.2

◆ **Question 13.4**
What pathology is present and how might this be related to the patient's death?

◆ **Question 13.5**
What clinical signs may have been present before death?

◆ **Question 13.6**
What investigation might have been used to confirm the diagnosis of mitral valve prolapse during life?

◆ **Question 13.7**
If severe mitral incompetence had been diagnosed during life what therapy might have been instituted?

Revision

■ Sudden death, see pp. 339–340

■ Mucoid degeneration of the mitral valve, see pp. 342–344

◆ **Answer 13.4**
There is mucoid degeneration of the mitral valve with marked billowing of the valve cusps (mitral valve prolapse). Such change may be present in 15% of subjects over the age of 70 years but in this case the change is severe and is occurring in a younger person. This lesion is associated with sudden cardiac death but the exact mechanism by which it causes death is unclear.

◆ **Answer 13.5**
Auscultation of the heart may have revealed a midsystolic click and a late cardiac murmur.

◆ **Answer 13.6**
Mitral valve prolapse is visualised easily by echocardiography.

◆ **Answer 13.7**
The mitral valve could have been replaced by a prosthetic device. This is likely to be required if the chordae tendineae rupture as may happen in the later stages of the process of mucoid degeneration.

Poor stream

A 70-year-old male patient presents to his general practitioner complaining of problems passing urine. The patient says that it is very difficult to start even though he badly needs to go. Even when he has passed urine he often feels that there is more to come but it does not. He frequently needs to micturate and is getting up two or three times in the night. This has been going on for several months getting slowly worse but what has caused him to present is the fact that even when he has urinated, he still continues to dribble urine and he finds this severely embarrassing. Added to this, the force with which he can urinate is very much reduced and it is difficult for him to avoid soiling his clothing.

◆ Question 14.1
What does this collection of symptoms suggest as a probable diagnosis?

The patient is put on the waiting list to see a urologist. He remains on the waiting list for some months repeatedly returning to the GP, complaining of worsening of clinical symptoms and developing a mild reactive depression for which he is treated with mild anxiolytics. He subsequently presents in Accident and Emergency in severe pelvic pain with inability to pass urine for the previous 24 hours.

◆ Question 14.2
What has now happened and how will it be treated as an emergency?

Following this emergency he is seen by the urologist who again examines the patient and recommends a preliminary biopsy and bone scan.

◆ Answer 14.1
This pattern of symptoms suggests urinary outflow obstruction. The likeliest cause of this in a male patient of this age is prostatic enlargement, although other conditions such as urinary calculi or bladder carcinoma should also enter the differential diagnosis. The enlarged prostate distorts the route of the urethra and compresses and lengthens it to as much as twice its normal length, this means that it can contain a reservoir of urine after micturition. In benign enlargement a median lobe develops and this can act as a ball valve restricting outflow resulting in difficulty in initiating micturition and in a poor stream. Behind this enlarged prostate urine may accumulate increasing the risk of stasis-related infection and calculus formation. The enlarged veins on the prostatic bed may cause mild haematuria at the beginning or end of micturition. Enlargement may be either benign or malignant.

◆ Answer 14.2
The patient has gone into acute retention. During this the patient is unable to pass any urine and the bladder distends painfully. Some patients with enlarged prostates may present in this way without any previous history of prostatic disease. In general, increased bladder pressure develops over some time and the muscles of the bladder wall hypertrophy forming trabeculations (Fig. 14.3). The areas between these may bulge out under the increased pressure, resulting in small sacculations or even the formation of a large bladder diverticulum. The emergency treatment is catheterization.

◆ Question 14.3
What does the urologist suspect and what aspect of the physical examination has led him to that suspicion?

The bone scan is negative and the pathology report describes 'an adequate core of prostatic tissue showing benign prostatic hyperplasia but no evidence of malignancy or atypia' (see Fig. 14.1). The patient is then admitted for surgery.

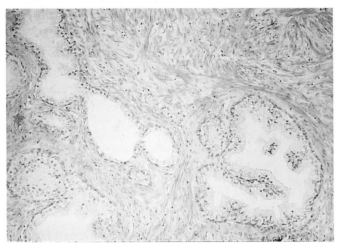

Fig. 14.1

◆ Question 14.4
What will the operation be?

Following surgery the pathology report describes foci of low-grade adenocarcinoma (see Fig. 14.2).

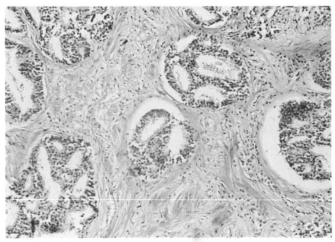

Fig. 14.2

◆ Answer 14.3
The most revealing aspect of the examination of the prostate is the rectal examination. The prostate can be felt through the rectal wall and a smooth, regular contour with preservation of the median sulcus is suggestive of benign disease. Since malignant disease begins as a focal mutation and clonal proliferation from this then the malignant prostate is likely to be irregular, the median sulcus may be destroyed and the organ feels hard and craggy. In this case the urologist felt that the patient's prostate was harder and more irregular than he would expect for benign disease although he was not certain that it was malignant. (Figure 14.3 shows benign prostatic hyperplasia.)

◆ Answer 14.4
A variety of operations are available to the surgeon but the most common is transurethral prostatectomy. In this operation an electric cautery device is passed into the bladder via the urethra and the prostate is cut into strips in situ. These are withdrawn through the urethra, placed in a suitable fixative (10% buffered formal saline is standard) and sent for histology. In many cases the volume of material is so great that it is impractical to examine it all and various sampling regimes (based on the weight of the sample) have been developed on the basis of the statistical chances of locating foci of cancer in large volumes of benign tissue. Some help is available from the fact that prostatic cancer is often yellow and hard compared with benign prostatic tissue.

◆ Question 14.5
Why is this different from the biopsy report?

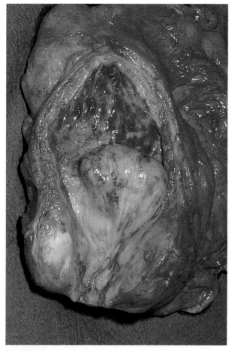

Fig. 14.3

It is agreed with the patient that he will undergo hormonal treatment and he remains symptom free until 4 years later when he is hospitalized for a stroke from which he dies 2 days later. The autopsy shows no evidence of metastatic carcinoma and the cause of death is given as:

> 1a Cerebrovascular accident
> 1b Hypertensive vascular disease.

◆ Question 14.6
Do you think that his prostatic carcinoma should appear on the OPCS cause of death?

Revision

■ Prostatic hyperplasia, see pp. 587–591

■ Prostatic carcinoma, see pp. 591–595

◆ Answer 14.5
An enlarged prostate may weigh many hundreds of grams and a core biopsy may weigh less than 1g, consequently there is a large risk of sampling error. Some surgeons may take multiple biopsies and some areas of the prostate are much more susceptible to malignant transformation than others. The term 'adequate' in the biopsy report refers to the technical adequacy of the specimen as a biopsy; it cannot refer to sampling adequacy and should not be interpreted in this way. The criteria for diagnosing cancer in prostatic biopsies are sometimes difficult to apply and if interpreted uncritically can lead to an unreasonably high rate of cancer diagnosis that far exceeds the known symptomatic rate.

◆ Answer 14.6
No. There is no evidence to suggest that either the prostatic carcinoma or its treatment contributed to the death and, therefore, it should not come under the section related to the direct cause of death (1a, 1b or 1c) and it cannot be said to have been a contributory cause unrelated to the major cause of death and, therefore, should not be entered under section 2. Section 2 is often incorrectly used to list other conditions that the patient had, but they should only be recorded here if they are a part of the *cause* of death.

Sir Walter Raleigh's disease

A 61-year-old delivery van driver goes to see his general practitioner in early summer complaining of a persistent cough. The patient is a lifelong cigarette smoker with an average consumption of 25 cigarettes/day. He says that he often has a cough in the winter months but not usually in the summer and that this cough has remained with him for 4 months. He brings up small amounts of redish sputum. On examination the GP finds that the man is reasonably fit with mild hypertension and obesity. On listening to his lungs there is decreased air entry into the left lung with a faint monophonic wheeze. The GP sends him to the local hospital for a chest radiograph which shows a shadow at the left hilum.

◆ **Question 15.1**
What is the most likely pathological cause of the shadow at the left hilum?

◆ **Question 15.2**
How might this diagnosis be confirmed?

Bronchoscopic biopsies confirm the diagnosis of squamous carcinoma and a thoracic surgeon removes the left lung at thoracotomy. Figure 15.1 shows the macroscopic appearances of the left lung.

◆ **Answer 15.1**
Given the patient's history, carcinoma of the lung is the most likely diagnosis.

◆ **Answer 15.2**
Cytology of sputum could confirm the presence of malignant cells but bronchoscopy would be required to locate the tumour and assess its operability and a tissue biopsy during this procedure would be the best method of confirming the diagnosis.

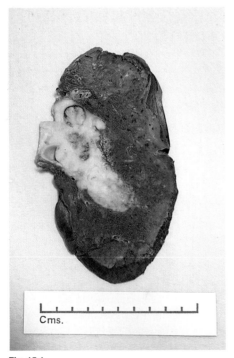

Cms.

Fig. 15.1

◆ **Question 15.3**
What is likely to be the physical basis of the monophonic wheeze heard on auscultation of the chest?

◆ **Question 15.4**
What changes are likely to be found in the lung tissue distal to the tumour?

◆ **Question 15.5**
What risk factors does this patient have for lung cancer?

The patient recovers from his operation and returns home. He attends for regular follow-up at the hospital and for the first few months his health is good. Nine months after the operation he complains of aches and pains in his legs and back and of thirst. The results of a blood test are:

	Patient's values	Normal range
Sodium	133 mmol/l	130–147 mmol/l
Potassium	4.1 mmol/l	3.3–5.5 mmol/l
Urea	6.2 mmol/l	3.3–8.3 mmol/l
Creatinine	115 μmol/l	60–120 μmol/l
Calcium	2.89 mmol/l	2.12–2.63 mmol/l

◆ **Question 15.6**
What abnormality is present and what might this be due to?

◆ **Question 15.7**
How might this diagnosis be confirmed?

Now that the tumour has spread to the patient's bones a cure is not possible but chemotherapy might produce some reduction in tumour size. The main care that the medical profession can offer is pain relief.

◆ **Answer 15.3**
Narrowing of the left main bronchus altering the pattern of airflow and producing the wheeze.

◆ **Answer 15.4**
An obstructive pneumonia due to narrowing of the main bronchus. Debris from this inflammatory process could have formed part of the sputum which the patient was expectorating together with material shed from the tumour itself.

◆ **Answer 15.5**
Cigarette smoking. There is a direct relationship between the number of cigarettes smoked and the risk of developing lung cancer. Other risk factors which are not present in this case include inhalation of asbestos fibres, inhalation of radioactive gases and industrial exposure to nickel, chromate, mustard gas or arsenic.

◆ **Answer 15.6**
The blood calcium level is raised. This could be due to the lung carcinoma giving rise to metastases in the bone, causing destruction of bone and release of calcium. The lung carcinoma could have produced a parathormone like substance causing resorption of bone and raising blood calcium but in this case the primary lung cancer has been removed so this is unlikely.

◆ **Answer 15.7**
Bony metastases could be visualised by plain radiographs or by bone scans.

◆ **Question 15.8**

What is the overall 5-year survival rate for carcinoma of the lung?

Revision

- Cytopathology, see pp. 68–70

- Carcinogenesis, see pp. 261–283

- Hypercalcaemia, see pp. 150, 515

- Lung carcinoma, see pp. 393–397

◆ **Answer 15.8**

5–7%. Only about 15% of cases are operable at the time of diagnosis and complete surgical resection is the only realistic chance of cure. Small-cell carcinoma of the lung has almost invariably metastasised by the time of presentation; although it may show some response to chemotherapy this treatment is rarely curative.

Fall onto an outstretched hand

You are a senior house officer in Accident and Emergency and are presented with a 7-year-old boy who has fallen onto his outstretched left hand. He is accompanied by his father who is angry and aggressive, the child is frightened and tearful. On examination the child has numerous bruises of different ages, one on his left shin, one on his forehead associated with a healing graze and one on the extensor surface of his right arm. There is a fresh graze on the palm of his left hand. There is a tender swelling on his left forearm and the arm seems to be bent upwards at an angle of about 15°. The child says that he fell off his new bicycle; the father is angry saying that the child has been playing the goat on the new cycle and doesn't deserve to have it, the child starts crying again, the father tells him not to be a baby.

◆ Question 16.1
What is the most important clinical thing to establish at this stage?

◆ Question 16.2
Given the information so far do you consider child abuse a possibility?

◆ Question 16.3
What radiographs would you take? What is this type of fracture called? How will you treat it?

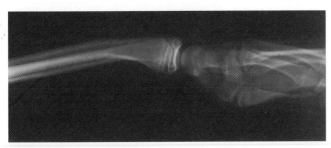

Fig. 16.1 X-ray prior to treatment

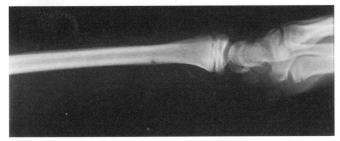

Fig. 16.2 X-ray following treatment

◆ Answer 16.1
In most bone injury situations the main cause of future problems is not the bone damage, but associated soft tissue damage; particularly nerve and vascular damage. Consequently pulses, sensory and motor function should be assessed and recorded at presentation and at all stages of treatment.

◆ Answer 16.2
Child abuse is always a possibility in child injury, but the pattern of injuries described is completely consistent with the history of a young child with or without a new cycle. The relationship between the child and his father is very common and shows a mixture of concern and guilt on the part of the father. In child abuse the child is generally younger and the pattern of injuries is often bizarre and inconsistent with the story of the injury.

◆ Answer 16.3
It is helpful to radiograph pairs of limbs of the young (Figs 16.1 and 16.2) since epiphyseal injuries, in particular, are best assessed against a normal control. This is a so-called 'greenstick' fracture in which the fracture involves only one cortical surface. As with most limb fractures the basis of therapy is reduction of the fracture and stabilization in some form of cast immobilizing both the joint above and the joint below the fracture. This allows callus to form at the fracture and to be remodelled as normal bone over a period of several weeks. Reduction of 'greenstick' fractures requires fracture of the unbroken cortical surface. This can be done under local anaesthetic, but it is wise to separate anxious parents from their offspring during this procedure.

◆ **Question 16.4**
Is this an adequate result? What is the most important clinical action at this time?

◆ **Question 16.5**
What types of injury might you expect in falls onto the outstretched hand in a healthy young adult or in an elderly osteoporotic woman?

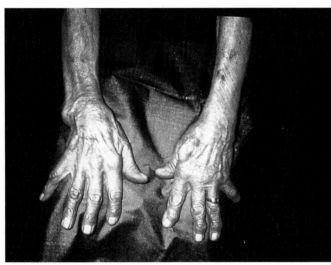

Fig. 16.3

Revision

■ Bone fractures and repair, see pp. 123–124, 785–787

■ Osteoporosis, see pp. 788–789

◆ **Answer 16.4**
This is a very good result. In the young a considerable degree of deformity will remodel since bone is an active tissue and is moulded by the active forces at work upon it, but it is preferable to get the best result possible at the first attempt. After reduction of the fracture and stabilisation, vascular and nervous integrity should again be assessed and recorded.

◆ **Answer 16.5**
In most adults you would not expect to see 'greenstick' fractures. Obviously the type of injury is going to depend upon the exact nature of the fall and the forces involved, but for falls from a standing position onto an outstretched hand a young adult might expect to fracture their clavicle rather than the much thicker and stronger forearm. Those animals such as dogs, cats and horses which routinely land on their forelimbs with considerable force, do not have clavicles. Young adults also have a tendency to fracture the scaphoid bone at the base of the thumb. This is an important fracture to recognize as the blood supply is distal and fracture can result in avascular necrosis with consequent instability of the thumb. In the elderly, often osteoporotic, human, the typical fracture from falls onto the outstretched hand produces a Colles' fracture. This involves the distal radius which is displaced dorsally and proximally giving a very characteristic clinical appearance (Fig. 16.3). The principles of therapy are again those aimed at giving callus and eventually mature bone the best chance of forming.

Breast mass

A 44-year-old woman notices a mass in her right breast. Her mother died of breast cancer at the age of 55, so the patient is very concerned about the lesion and presents to her general practitioner the next day. Her GP notes a firm mobile 15-mm diameter mass in the upper outer quadrant of the right breast. He examines her thoroughly and there are no other abnormal physical signs. The case notes show that she had an area of cervical intraepithelial neoplasia, grade 3, treated by laser at the age of 40; she has been discharged from follow-up.

◆ Question 17.1
What are the most likely explanations for the mass?

One week later the patient is seen by a general surgeon in his outreach clinic in the Fund-Holding GP's surgery. He notes that the mass is highly mobile, is not fixed to skin or underlying muscle, that the axillary lymph nodes are not enlarged, and that the nipple is not retracted (Fig. 17.1).

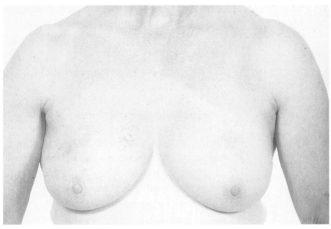

Fig. 17.1

◆ Question 17.2
What options are available to the surgeon for diagnosing the breast mass?

◆ Question 17.3
What are the arguments for and against each of these methods?

◆ Answer 17.1
The most likely explanations are:

- breast cancer
- fibroadenoma
- fibrocystic disease.

Cervical intraepithelial neoplasia is not invasive and so does not metastasise. Even if the cervical lesion had been invasive, squamous carcinoma metastasising to the breast is exceptionally rare.

◆ Answer 17.2
The surgeon could request mammography (radiographic examination of the breast), perform fine-needle aspiration cytology, a Tru-Cut biopsy, or an intraoperative frozen section.

◆ Answer 17.3

- Mammography would not necessarily give a definite diagnosis and is less successful in patients under 50 as younger patients have more opaque appearing breast making lesions difficult to visualise. If performed it should always *precede* needle biopsy because any resulting haematoma reduces sensitivity of the examination.
- Fine-needle aspiration cytology is the method of choice for diagnosis of breast lesions. It is relatively painless, rapid, sensitive and specific for carcinoma.
- Cutting needle biopsy is an alternative when no cytology service is available, or when FNAC has produced on unsatisfactory aspirate. Even with local anaesthesia it can be uncomfortable, may produce a haematoma, and may miss the

(contd)

The surgeon performs the procedure shown in Figure 17.2.

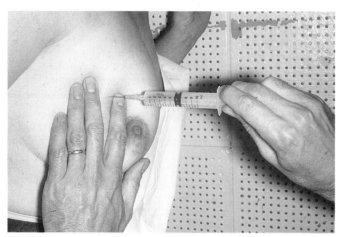

Fig. 17.2

◆ **Question 17.4**
What is shown in Figure 17.2?

The patient's cytological preparation is shown in Figure 17.3. The report reads: 'This is a good aspirate of large branching clumps of benign epithelial cells typical of a fibroadenoma. No malignant cells are seen.'

The surgeon reassures the patient in outpatients the next week that the lump is benign and could be left unoperated. The patient, concerned about the fate which befell her mother requests excision.

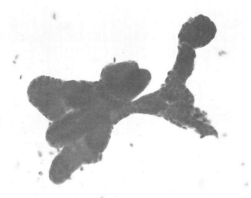

Fig 17.3

lesion especially where, like this one, it is very mobile. There is some evidence that the modern spring-loaded cutting needles, such as 'Biopty-cut', which leave one of the operator's hands free to fix the lesion being biopsied, produce more accurate biopsies than 'Tru-cut' needles which required both hands to operate them.
- Frozen section diagnosis is going out of favour. The patient faces what many consider an ordeal of submitting to an operation, the extent of which is to be determined while she is anaesthetized. Even if the lesion is shown to be carcinoma, surgery more radical than just removing the mass completely may not be necessary. Frozen sections have a significant false negative rate due mainly to sampling error. There is even a false positive rate for the diagnosis of cancer of around 1:1000.

◆ **Answer 17.4**
This is fine-needle aspiration cytology. The skin may be anaesthetized first, then a fine needle of similar gauge to that used for venepuncture is passed into the lesion several times while the operator sucks with a 20-ml syringe. The syringe and needle are then rinsed out into 5 ml of transport fluid which is taken to the cytopathology laboratory.

◆ Question 17.5
Are her fears justified?

In view of her concerns the surgeon performs an excision biopsy of the lesion the next week as a day case procedure. The patient makes a good recovery with no additional problems. The histopathology report confirms the cytological diagnosis of fibroadenoma, but also mentions foci of lobular carcinoma-in-situ (Fig. 17.4) without invasion in the adjacent breast tissue.

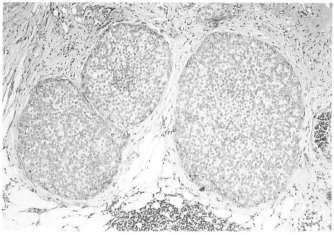

Fig 17.4

◆ Question 17.6
What is the significance for the patient of finding lobular carcinoma-in-situ?

◆ Question 17.7
What action should the surgeon take and why?

In the UK, quite apart from her history of breast disease, the patient will be invited to attend every 3 years for breast screening mammography from age 50. The surgeon arranges regular mammograms up to the age of 50 and advises the patient to take advantage of the breast screening programme when she reaches 50.

Revision

- Cytopathology, see pp. 68–70
- Biopsy, see p. 533
- Carcinoma of the breast, see pp. 536–550
- Breast screening, see p. 528

◆ Answer 17.5
The lesion is most unlikely to be malignant, but her general worries are well founded. Although the overall breast cancer rate for women in the United Kingdom is about 1:12, this rises to 1:2 when two first degree relatives have developed the disease. Family history is one of the most important risk factors.

◆ Answer 17.6
The presence of lobular carcinoma-in-situ signifies a 10 times increased risk for developing subsequent invasive breast cancer compared with unaffected patients.

◆ Answer 17.7
The increased risk of invasive cancer applies to both breasts, not just the one in which the lobular carcinoma-in-situ has been detected. Therefore the only logical operation to perform if one were chosen would be bilateral simple mastectomy. In the UK, most surgeons recommend careful follow-up to their patients, possibly with mammography to increase the chance of detecting early abnormalities.

CASE 18

'I'm exhausted!'

A 40-year-old mother of 4 children (girls 16, 13, 10 and boy 18 years old), attends her general practitioner's (GP) surgery. When asked what the problem is she replies 'I'm exhausted!'.

◆ Question 18.1
Although this presentation is vague, what possibilities should be considered initially?

The patient says that she finds her family commitments a burden, particularly coping with the two older daughters who are always quarrelling, but the feeling of tiredness and exhaustion does not seem to be related. When asked about any other symptoms she replies that she 'gets out of breath easily' and has been constipated recently with episodes of abdominal pain. She says she hasn't had time to weigh herself, but she thinks she has lost weight. Her periods are normal. The GP notices that the patient looks pale and depressed.

◆ Question 18.2
What conclusions do you draw from these observations?

On examination, there are no abnormal findings in neurological examination or on examination of the cardiovascular or respiratory systems. In the abdomen, however, there is a soft vague mass in the right iliac fossa, but she is constipated and this is interpreted as faeces in the caecum and ascending colon. The GP takes a blood sample for haemoglobin estimation and, having assumed that the patient has anaemia and that it is due to iron deficiency, prescribes ferrous sulphate 120 mg daily. For her constipation, liquid paraffin is prescribed.

Three days later the laboratory confirms that she is anaemic: the haemoglobin is 9 g/dl. A week later the patient returns feeling very unwell. She now has diarrhoea and what she says are 'piles'. The GP refers her to a consultant physician at the local hospital.

◆ Question 18.3
What gastrointestinal disorders could be responsible for the patient's signs and symptoms?

The gastroenterologist takes a full history and examines the patient. He finds no evidence of haemorrhoids, but notices that the anus is rather inflamed; he attributes this to the recent diarrhoea. He suspects that the patient has coeliac disease (gluten-sensitive enteropathy).

◆ Question 18.4
What investigations should be performed?

◆ Answer 18.1
Assuming that the feeling of exhaustion is a new and persistent problem for the patient, the possibilities include social, psychiatric and organic conditions. The GP needs to find out whether there has been a change in her domestic or personal circumstances placing her under greater strain or if there is evidence of an illness.

◆ Answer 18.2
The shortness of breath and the skin pallor would be consistent with anaemia. The constipation may have no diagnostic significance, but the possibility of a gastrointestinal disorder should be considered. Weight loss, if proven, is a worrying feature of any illness, but does not necessarily mean that the cause is an alimentary disorder. However, the next thing to do is examine the patient.

◆ Answer 18.3
Gastrointestinal disorders often present with or are complicated by anaemia. Iron deficiency anaemia is often due to chronic blood loss from the surface of ulcers in the stomach or duodenum or from tumours anywhere in the gut. Haemorrhoids ('piles') may also bleed causing anaemia if recurrent or persistent. Anaemia due to vitamin B_{12} deficiency may be caused by either autoimmune gastritis with loss of intrinsic factor (pernicious anaemia) or disease affecting the site of absorption of the B_{12} intrinsic factor complex. Folate deficiency is common in diseases causing intestinal malabsorption.

◆ Answer 18.4
The most useful investigation will be histological examination of a duodenal or jejunal mucosal biopsy. The type of anaemia should also be identified.

The patient has a blood sample taken for haematological and biochemical analysis, and agrees to attend the next endoscopy clinic for biopsy of her duodenum.

The laboratory findings on the blood sample are:

	Patient's values	Normal range
Haemoglobin	9.2 g/dl	11.5–15.5 g/dl
Red cell count	2.8×10^{12}/litre	$4.5–6.5 \times 10^{12}$/litre
Mean cell volume (MCV)	65 fl	80–95 fl
Albumin	3.0 g/l	35–50 g/l

Abnormally numerous reticulocytes are noted on a blood film.

The duodenal biopsy has the appearances shown in Figure 18.1.

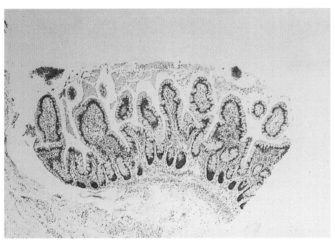

Fig. 18.1

◆ Question 18.5
What is your interpretation of these findings?

The patient sees the gastroenterologist a week later for the results. She is told that she doesn't have coeliac disease, but is still anaemic and should continue with the iron tablets. Her condition is unchanged. She is still exhausted, troubled by bouts of diarrhoea and constipation, and still worried that she has 'piles'. Examination of the abdomen reveals a slightly tender mass in the right iliac fossa which couldn't be felt on the last visit.

The gastroenterologist advises the patient to be admitted to hospital for investigation, firstly for a colonoscopy. This shows areas of mucosal reddening in the rectum and descending colon; biopsies are taken (Fig. 18.2).

◆ Answer 18.5
The patient is still anaemic. The MCV and mean cell haemoglobin concentration (MCHC) are both low, consistent with iron deficiency. The reticulocyte count is high, probably due to a combination of response to iron therapy and continued internal blood loss. The duodenal biopsy is normal; it bears long villi and virtually excludes coeliac disease (in which the villi would be atrophic).

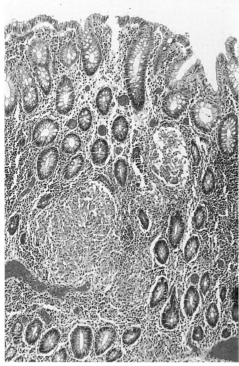

Fig 18.2

◆ **Question 18.6**
What does the biopsy show and what is the most likely diagnosis?

◆ **Question 18.7**
What should be done next?

The barium examination reveals narrowing of the terminal ileum consistent with Crohn's disease.

◆ **Question 18.8**
How should the patient be treated?

The patient feels better within days of starting treatment. She returns home. By 6 weeks after discharge from hospital, her haemoglobin has risen to 13 g/dl, her bowel actions are normal, and she doesn't feel unduly exhausted.

◆ **Answer 18.6**
The biopsy shows granulomas in the lamina propria of the colonic mucosa. While the presence of granulomas in any biopsy raises the possibility of a mycobacterial infection (e.g. tuberculosis), this is very unlikely in the large bowel. The diagnosis is probably Crohn's disease. The colonoscopic appearances suggesting patchy rather than continuous inflammation are consistent with this diagnosis. The anal inflammation, possibly with fissures or a fistula, is common in Crohn's disease and may also be found to contain granulomas if biopsied.

◆ **Answer 18.7**
Because Crohn's disease most commonly involves the small bowel, particularly the terminal ileum, it is necessary to determine the extent of the disease in this patient. This is done by radiological examination of the abdomen after ingestion of barium.

◆ **Answer 18.8**
Crohn's disease is now rarely treated by surgery initially. The patient is put on a low-fat, low-fibre diet and prescribed 20 mg prednisolone daily.

◆ **Question 18.9**

What is the prognosis?

Revision

■ Anaemia, see pp. 685, 699–722

■ Chronic granulomatous inflammation, see pp. 237, 241–244

■ Crohn's disease, see pp. 431–435

◆ **Answer 18.9**   VARIES

Crohn's disease is a chronic relapsing inflammatory disorder of unknown aetiology. There is, therefore, no specific treatment and no patient can be regarded as cured even if their initial symptoms and signs have disappeared. Approximately 80% of patients eventually require surgery to deal with fistulas or obstructing strictures or failure to respond to medical treatment. Half of the cases treated surgically will develop further recurrences.

Tiredness and headaches

A 56-year-old man comes to your general practitioner's surgery complaining of tiredness and headaches. Over the last year this has been getting steadily worse; now he is struggling to carry on his work as a builder.

On examination he is pale, slightly thin (he admits on further questioning to have lost about 8 kg over the last year) and has two ballottable masses in the loins which move with respiration. His blood pressure is 180/100.

◆ Question 19.1
What are the masses likely to be?

You immediately refer the patient to a urological surgeon for investigation of the masses. You suspect that the hypertension could be related to them.

◆ Question 19.2
Why?

◆ Question 19.3
What are the treatable causes of hypertension?

The urologist examines the patient and confirms your impression. The patient's blood biochemistry shows high potassium, urea, creatinine and phosphate together with low albumin.

◆ Question 19.4
What do these indicate?

The patient's full blood count shows normochromic normocytic anaemia.

◆ Question 19.5
What does this indicate?

The hospital confirms the diagnosis of adult type polycystic renal disease by ultrasound of the kidneys. Since there is no treatment available, the hypertension is managed by drugs and the renal failure by dietary restrictions.

◆ Question 19.6
What genetic advice should the patient be given?

◆ Answer 19.1
They are most likely to be renal masses in view of the position and movement with respiration.

◆ Answer 19.2
The masses might be polycystic kidneys, which are a cause of hypertension.

◆ Answer 19.3
These include renal failure, renal artery stenosis, polycystic kidneys, raised intracranial pressure, endocrine lesions such as phaeochromocytoma, Cushing's disease and syndrome, acromegaly and (where appropriate) toxaemia of pregnancy.

◆ Answer 19.4
These are the typical biochemical findings of chronic renal failure.

◆ Answer 19.5
This is the 'anaemia of chronic disorders', a finding common in chronic conditions such as chronic renal failure.

◆ Answer 19.6
Adult polycystic disease is inherited as an autosomal dominant condition with high penetrance. In practice this means that just under half of his children will develop the disease.

One year later the patient is readmitted from outpatients. He has severe headaches, is drowsy and is complaining of a painful finger (Fig. 19.1). His blood pressure is 210/130.

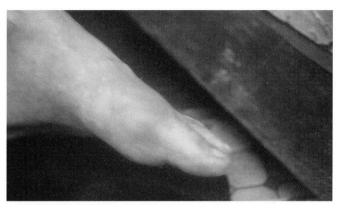

Fig. 19.1

◆ **Question 19.7**
What is the most likely explanation for these findings?

The patient's renal failure is brought under control by haemodialysis, but his hypertension remains unmanageable. The surgeon explains the need for bilateral nephrectomy to the patient: the kidneys will never work again and are causing his hypertension which must be controlled urgently. Congenital berry aneurysms, which can cause subarachnoid haemorrhage, are associated with polycystic kidneys.

Figure 19.2 shows one of the patient's nephrectomy specimens. Figure 19.3 is the medium power histological appearance in the surviving parenchyma between the cysts.

◆ **Answer 19.7**
He probably has hypertensive encephalopathy due to end-stage renal failure. The gouty tophi on his finger are due to sodium urate accumulation in chronic renal failure.

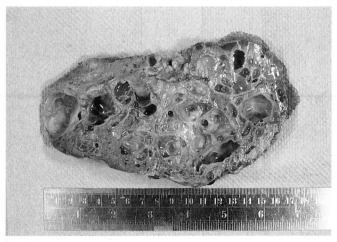

Fig. 19.2

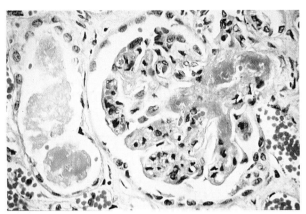

Fig. 19.3

◆ Question 19.8
What do these show?

The patient was maintained on haemodialysis for 2 years and then had a successful kidney transplant from a motor cyclist with fatal head injuries.

Revision

■ Renal cystic disease, see pp. 624–626

■ Hypertension, see pp. 319–324

■ Anaemia, see pp. 699–722

■ Inheritance of genetic disorders, see p. 45

◆ Answer 19.8
The kidney (Fig. 19.2) shows multiple parenchymal cysts of varying sizes typical of polycystic renal disease. Between these, histology (Fig. 19.3) reveals fibrinoid necrosis of the afferent arteriole of the glomerulus shown. This indicates accelerated phase hypertension.

Glycosuria and a rash

A 60-year-old woman has been referred to your medical out-patient clinic with a 2 month history of polyuria and weight loss. The general practitioner has performed urine tests and found the patient to have glycosuria.

◆ **Question 20.1**
What are the likely causes of glycosuria in a patient with this history?

◆ **Question 20.2**
What are the causes of secondary diabetic states?

The patient arrives and she immediately tells you that she has developed a rash in the 3 weeks that she has been waiting for her clinic appointment. The rash has been variably distributed over her body and is getting worse. Your history taking reveals nothing else of note.

On examination, you notice that she has a rash around her mouth, (Fig. 20.1) on her face and on her trunk.

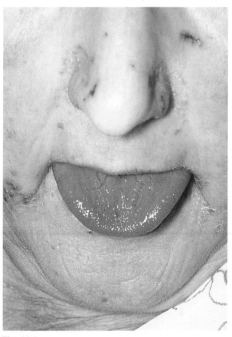

Fig. 20.1

◆ **Question 20.3**
What kind of rash is shown in Figure 20.1?

◆ **Answer 20.1**
The patient is likely to have hyperglycaemia leading to the glycosuria. This is likely to be due either to diabetes mellitus of the type I (insulin-dependant) type, which would be unusual in a patient of this age, or to secondary diabetes, that is to say a diabetic state resulting from another medical disorder. Maturity onset (type II) diabetes mellitus, while common in this age group, is associated with *excess* weight rather than weight loss.

◆ **Answer 20.2**
These are all due to excess of hormones having a hyperglycaemic effect. The conditions therefore include: glucagonoma, somatostatinoma, phaeochromocytoma, acromegaly and Cushing's disease and syndrome.

◆ **Answer 20.3**
This is an erythematous rash with epidermal necrosis. The differential diagnosis of the rash includes erythema multiforme, the blistering disorders (pemphigoid and pemphigus) and one very rare condition.

As a consultant endocrinologist, you remember reading about cases of glucagonoma of the pancreas being associated with a rare skin rash called necrolytic migratory erythema.

◆ Question 20.4
What should you do at this stage?

The patient's blood tests show marked hyperglycaemia (glucose 22 mmol L^{-1}) associated with elevated blood glucagon levels. The skin biopsy result is consistent with necrolytic migratory erythema. The patient's skin now looks like Figure 20.2. The patient has no abnormalities on abdominal examination.

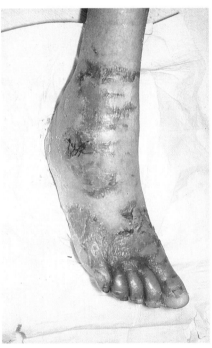

Fig. 20.2

◆ Answer 20.4
The patient's rash is serious, whatever the exact diagnosis, and she needs urgent endocrinological work-up, so she should be admitted to hospital. She needs her blood biochemistry testing, including assay of all the hormones which can cause hyperglycaemia and a dermatological opinion on her skin rash supported by a biopsy for exact histological diagnosis.

◆ Question 20.5
What test should be done now?

The patient's CT scan shows a mass in the tail of the pancreas. You arrange angiograms which show a highly vascular mass in the pancreas consistent with an endocrine neoplasm. The veins leading from the mass contain vastly elevated levels of glucagon.

◆ Question 20.6
Why does the patient need these invasive procedures?

The patient's distal pancreatectomy specimen is shown in Figure 20.3.

◆ Answer 20.5
A computerised tomography (CT) scan of the abdomen would be a good investigation to look for masses in the pancreas.

◆ Answer 20.6
The mass imaged in the pancreas may not be making the appropriate hormone. You need to know for sure that distal pancreatectomy would remove the source of hormone, as it is a difficult procedure with a significant mortality.

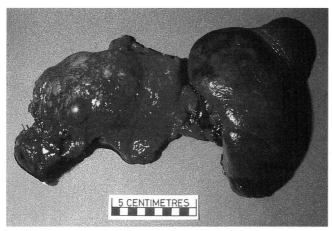

Fig. 20.3

◆ Question 20.7
What can you see?

Figure 20.4 shows the pancreatic tumour stained by the immunoperoxidase technique for glucagon.

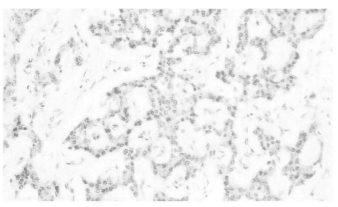

Fig. 20.4

◆ Question 20.8
What is the purpose of this special stain?

After the major surgery the patient eventually made a good recovery: her secondary diabetes and the skin rash rapidly subsided. Her prognosis is uncertain because although the majority of glucagonomas are benign they are unpredictable in behaviour, in common with all other islet cell tumours of the pancreas.

Revision
- Diabetes, see pp. 518–520
- Pancreatic islet tumours, see pp. 520–521

◆ Answer 20.7
There is a rounded mass in the pancreas.

◆ Answer 20.8
This stain is dependant upon antibodies to glucagon binding to glucagon in the tissue section. The antibodies have an enzyme bound to them which leads to a chemical reaction resulting in a brown colour where they have bound. The brown colour of most of the cells in Figure 20.4 indicates that they contain glucagon.

CASE 21

Change in a mole

A 20-year-old woman presents to her general practitioner with a mole on her left shoulder. The woman says it has changed recently, itches and has bled slightly.

On examination the appearances are those seen in Figure 21.1. The lesion is nodular, 0.9 mm diameter, with a satellite nodule, the border is irregular and inflamed, the pigmentation is varied. The GP takes a diagnostic incisional biopsy under local anaesthetic and sends it for histology.

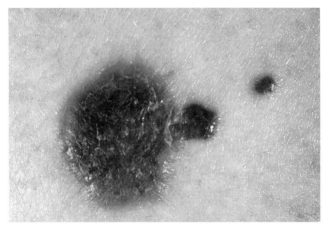

Fig. 21.1

◆ Question 21.1
Do you agree with the GP's management so far?

◆ Question 21.2
What is your differential diagnosis at this stage?

The lesion is excised fully. The histology of the excision specimen is shown in Figure 21.2.

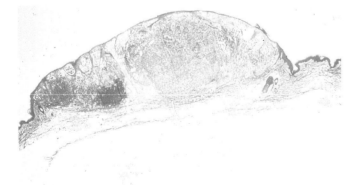

Fig. 21.2

◆ Answer 21.1
No. If a malignant melanoma is suspected then an urgent referral to a dermatologist is the correct management. The average GP is unlikely to see more than one melanoma every 2 years and cannot be expected to be confident about them. An incisional biopsy, which only samples the tumour, may make subsequent assessment and prognostication difficult, and there is the theoretical risk of inducing dissemination. The treatment of choice is full excision with a clear surgical margin.

◆ Answer 21.2
At this stage malignant melanoma is the most likely diagnosis. A benign pigmented naevus (particularly a Spitz naevus) is a possibility. Another, less likely, diagnosis includes basal cell papilloma (seborrheic wart).

◆ **Question 21.3**

What information would be on the histology report?

◆ **Question 21.4**

What is the next step in clinical management?

The patient is discharged back to the GP. Three months later she returns complaining of a new nodule at the original site. On examination she has multiple nodules in the skin and enlarged lymph nodes. She is referred back to the hospital.

◆ **Question 21.5**

What has happened to the patient?

◆ **Question 21.6**

What is the next line of treatment?

After her course of treatment she returns home. Three weeks later she becomes jaundiced and passes black urine.

◆ **Question 21.7**

What has developed now?

She is readmitted to hospital where she claims that all her symptoms are due to acquired immunodeficiency syndrome (AIDS) contracted whilst working as a prostitute. Her family deny the possibility of this being true. A psychiatric opinion is sought; the psychiatrist says that the condition is 'organic'.

◆ **Question 21.8**

What has happened?

As she is being prepared for chemotherapy she has a cardiac dysrhythmia and a fatal cardiac arrest. No attempt is made at resuscitation.

◆ **Answer 21.3**

Malignant melanoma, with Pagetoid spread. Maximum depth 1.3 mm but excision is incomplete.

◆ **Answer 21.4**

It is essential that the lesion is completely excised; this includes the lateral and deep margins of the tumour with a surround of normal tissue. A 50 mm margin of normal tissue with subsequent skin grafting used to be recommended, but there is no evidence that this improves survival and the cosmetic disfigurement is considerable. Some surgeons recommend prophylactic lymph node resection or perfusion with chemotherapeutic agents (at appropriate sites) but there is no evidence that this affects survival either.

◆ **Answer 21.5**

A recurrence at the original site may be due to incomplete primary removal or to metastasis from circulating malignant cells. Metastatic disease can arise after many years of apparently disease-free survival.

◆ **Answer 21.6**

Many chemotherapeutic regimes are undergoing trials at the moment, but none have been found to increase survival although they may help to control local disease. Local surgery and radiotherapy can also be used to control local disease.

◆ **Answer 21.7**

Some patients develop such a large tumour load that circulating melanin levels can colour the urine. The liver is a common site for metastases and obstructive jaundice often develops.

◆ **Answer 21.8**

'Organic' psychoses are distinguished from 'functional' psychoses by the presence of some demonstrable

(contd)

◆ **Question 21.9**
Do you agree with this clinical decision not to resuscitate this patient?

An autopsy is requested to determine the extent of disease. The relatives agree.

◆ **Question 21.10**
What significant sites of metastasis are revealed?

Fig. 21.3 Horizontal slice of the brain at post-mortem showing secondary melanoma deposits.

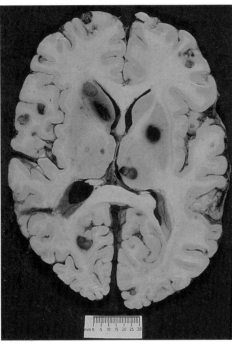

Fig. 21.3

physical cause such as drug intoxication, infections, degenerative diseases or, as in this case, tumours metastatic to the brain. Fits, convulsions and 'strokes' can also be the consequences of metastatic disease; they may be the presenting signs in many cases.

◆ **Answer 21.9**
It is a difficult medical ethical problem to know when to withhold active treatment, but most people would agree that in terminal care it would be inappropriate to resuscitate someone.

◆ **Answer 21.10**
The autopsy reveals widespread metastatic disease with deposits in the lymph nodes, liver, intestines, brain and heart as well as widespread skin involvement. It is said that metastases can be found in the heart in 80% of deaths from carcinomatosis. This patient was on a drug trial and it was noted that even small deposits of tumour had necrotic centres suggesting that although the drug regime had not cured the patient, there had been some effect and manipulations of dosage, timing and combinations with other drugs might be more effective.

Revision

■ Melanocytic skin lesions, see pp. 769–773

■ Metastasis, see pp. 251, 184–287

■ Cerebral metastases, see p. 872

■ Autopsy, see pp. 75–76

Painful joints

A 59-year-old man presents to his general practitioner with a recent history of a painful right knee. The man does not associate it with any specific trauma and he finds it difficult to describe the pain and to localize it accurately. In the past he has played a lot of squash and tennis but gave them up a few years previously as his performance began to deteriorate. He also found that his right hip ached after strenuous games and sometimes kept him awake at nights. On examination he had a restricted range of hip movements, flexion and abduction being particularly affected in the right hip. No restriction to movement was found in the knees.

◆ Question 22.1
What is the differential diagnosis?

◆ Question 22.2
What investigations would you perform?

◆ Question 22.3
What is the likely cause of his knee pains?

He is given mild analgesics and recommended to use these, particularly if joint pains disturb sleep. He returns 3 years later complaining that both the right hip and knee are constantly painful and limit both his walking and sleeping severely. He is examined again and this shows progression of his disease and limitations of movement in both hips.

◆ Question 22.4
What does the radiograph show? (Fig. 22.1).

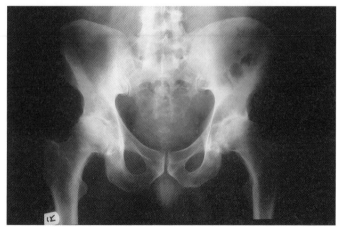

Fig. 22.1

◆ Answer 22.1
Arthropathies are common diseases and include a variety of pathogenic mechanisms. They may be primary, such as osteoarthrosis (osteoarthritis) which is non-inflammatory, tends to affect large joints, is often monoarticular and seems to be associated with 'wear and tear', or they may be associated with multisystem disease such as rheumatoid disease, in which case they may be inflammatory, affect small joints, are symmetrical in distribution and of obscure autoimmune pathogenesis. Arthropathies can occur as the result of infection, crystal deposition, tumours, trauma or as part of another disease such as psoriasis or chronic inflammatory bowel disease.

◆ Answer 22.2
This is a very good history of osteoarthrosis (osteoarthritis) and radiographs should be confirmatory although symptoms may precede any marked radiological changes. Infectious causes would be associated with clinical symptoms (such as obvious inflammation of the joint) and an increased white cell count while rheumatoid disease is commonly associated with rheumatoid factor (IgA-IgM complexes) in the blood.

◆ Answer 22.3
Quite commonly the most uncomfortable aspect of the condition is referred pain, often to the knee or lower leg. When the hip is treated the knee pain generally disappears.

◆ Answer 22.4
The hip radiograph (Fig. 22.1) shows narrowing of the joint space, osteophyte formation and some cystic change in the bone and if the patient has become inactive then there may be secondary osteopaenia (osteoporosis).

◆ **Question 22.5**
What treatment will you recommend?

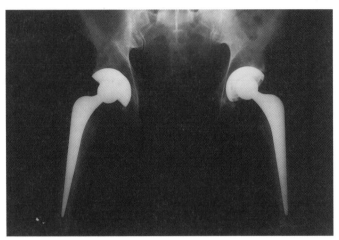

Fig. 22.2

◆ **Question 22.6**
What will the surgical specimen show? Two months later at surgical outpatients his thumbs show the features seen in Figure 22.3, what are these?

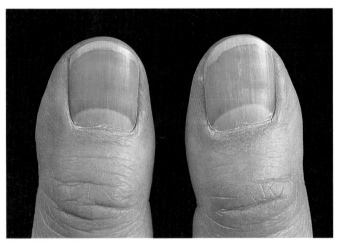

Fig. 22.3

Following surgery the patient mobilises well and the problems in his hips abate. Seven years later he stumbles on a kerbstone twisting the right hip. Following this he has progressively worsening pain and instability in the right hip and he is again referred to the orthopaedic surgeons. His new symptoms also include pain at the base of both thumbs.

◆ **Answer 22.5**
There is no effective medical treatment except for analgesia. Although there is no primary inflammation, secondary inflammation and surrounding muscle pain may be alleviated with non-steroidal anti-inflammatory drugs. Eventually, when the condition becomes disabling and the patient will no longer tolerate the discomfort then surgical replacement of the head of femur and the acetabular cup provides very significant improvement (Fig. 22.2). The reason for delay, particularly in young patients, is that the lifetime of a hip replacement is about 10 to 20 years on average.

◆ **Answer 22.6**
The specimen of the head of femur showed eburnation and remodelling of the joint surface, osteophytes around the lateral margin, subchondral bone cysts and sclerosis of the bone. The nail grooves are Beau's lines and represent areas of disturbed growth which may occur following any severe systemic trauma such as surgery, cytotoxic drugs, measles, mumps, pneumonia, coronary artery thrombosis or episodes of ingestion of toxic compounds such as arsenic (when they are called Mee's lines).

◆ **Question 22.7**

What has happened and what will the surgeons recommend? Are the pains in his thumbs likely to be related to his other problems?

After surgery he is well and active and dies of a myocardial infarction whilst out walking on his eighty-fifth birthday.

Revision

■ Osteoarthritis (osteoarthrosis), see pp. 803–805

■ Joint disorders, see pp. 802–817

■ Inflammation, see pp. 221–244

◆ **Answer 22.7**

Prosthesis failure often follows trauma to the joint. The prosthesis becomes loosened in the cement which allows in fluid and particles which wear away the contact surfaces releasing more particles and letting in more fluid until the whole structure becomes intolerably unstable. The original surgery can be repeated and although second replacements are not as statistically satisfactory as the initial ones, the results are good enough to make the surgery worthwhile.

Another preferred site for osteoarthrosis is at the base of the thumbs.

An epidemic

A 14-year-old schoolgirl at a single-sex boarding school feels unwell 2 weeks after the start of the autumn term. The school doctor is asked to see her. The pupil complains of nausea and malaise. The doctor finds nothing abnormal on routine examination, but notes that during the summer vacation she had been on a camping holiday to Spain with her parents. The doctor advises her to rest.

One month later, four other pupils become similarly unwell.

◆ Question 23.1
Could these illnesses be related?

The school nurse reports to the doctor that one of the girls appears jaundiced and routine urine testing reveals excess bilirubin in her urine. None of the others is jaundiced.

◆ Question 23.2
Could all these girls have viral hepatitis?

The doctor takes blood samples from all five girls and sends the samples for testing for antibodies to hepatitis viruses and for liver biochemistry. The liver biochemistry results in the four new cases show marked elevation of the serum transaminases, bilirubin concentration either at or slightly above the upper limit of the normal range, but only slight elevation of the alkaline phosphatase. All five samples contain an antibody to hepatitis A virus (HAV).

◆ Question 23.3
What is the diagnostic significance of the liver biochemistry results?

◆ Question 23.4
What further information is required about the HAV antibodies?

The antibodies to the hepatitis A virus are IgM class in each of the five girls. The infection has probably been imported by the first girl who picked up the virus during her camping holiday in Spain. The incubation period is typically 2–7 weeks, which fits with the history of the epidemic. The doctor advises the school administration that the girls should be segregated from the rest of the school until the risk of infection has passed.

During the next 3 weeks there are two further cases. Only one of the cases become jaundiced, but they all make a full recovery and return to their studies.

◆ Answer 23.1
Yes. Whenever large numbers of people share accommodation, especially if they are children encountering new pathogens for the first time, there is a risk of epidemics.

◆ Answer 23.2
Yes. Most people who develop viral hepatitis do not become jaundiced (so-called 'anicteric hepatitis'). In fact, many people with antibodies to hepatitis A virus do not have a known medical history of hepatitis (so-called 'subclinical hepatitis').

◆ Answer 23.3
The combination of marked elevation of serum transaminases with only slight elevation of the alkaline phosphatase strongly indicates hepatocellular injury ('hepatic jaundice') rather than biliary obstruction ('post-hepatic jaundice'); in 'pre-hepatic jaundice', such as that due to haemolysis, the liver biochemistry would be normal apart from a raised bilirubin.

◆ Answer 23.4
To distinguish between a very recent infection and longstanding immunity, the class of the antibody should be determined. IgG class HAV antibodies denote longstanding immunity, whereas IgM class HAV antibodies are evidence of very recent infection.

◆ Question 23.5
Shouldn't the doctor have arranged for the cases to have a liver biopsy to prove the diagnosis and to see how severely affected the livers were?

Fifteen years later, our patient, now aged 29, is referred by her family doctor for investigation of infertility. After leaving school, she trained as a nurse and, at the age of 24, married a journalist. She and her husband have been trying to start a family; 2 years ago she became pregnant, but had a miscarriage at 8 weeks. Her menstrual periods are irregular.

◆ Question 23.6
What disorders are associated with infertility?

The patient and her husband are thoroughly investigated. The husband's sperm count is normal. Investigation of the patient's pelvic organs reveals no abnormality. Careful clinical examination, however, reveals slight hepatomegaly. Liver biochemistry is performed revealing:

	Patient's values	Normal range
Alanine aminotransferase (ALT)	80 U/l	5–40 U/l
Alkaline phosphatase	350 U/l	30–110 U/l
Albumin	35 g/l	35–50 g/l
Bilirubin	22 μmol/l	5–17 μmol/l

◆ Question 23.7
What is the implication of these findings?

The patient is referred to a hepatologist. Further investigations are performed including testing for auto-antibodies which reveals anti-smooth muscle antibody and anti-nuclear factor.

◆ Question 23.8
What is the diagnosis?

Liver biopsy is performed, histology of which shows expansion of portal tracts by inflammation and fibrosis, foci of active piecemeal necrosis and swelling of hepatocytes. The architecture is not cirrhotic. These appearances are entirely consistent with autoimmune 'lupoid' hepatitis in a pre-cirrhotic phase.

◆ Question 23.9
What is the relationship between the earlier episode of viral hepatitis and the patient's current problem?

◆ Answer 23.5
No. Recovery from the acute illness is good in the vast majority of cases and the admittedly small risk of liver biopsy could not be justified.

◆ Answer 23.6
Infertility may be due to disorders of the male or female partner. In females, infertility may be caused by disease of the internal genitalia or systemic disorders. Systemic disorders causing infertility may be endocrine or non-endocrine.

◆ Answer 23.7
The patient clearly has active liver disease. The biochemistry is more consistent with a hepatitic process than with biliary disease.

◆ Answer 23.8
Probably autoimmune 'lupoid' hepatitis, an autoimmune variety of chronic liver disease in which the targets for immune injury are the hepatocytes.

◆ Answer 23.9
Probably none. An episode of viral hepatitis may cause someone with asymptomatic chronic liver disease to seek medical attention, but hepatitis A rarely progresses to chronic liver disease.

The patient is told that she has chronic liver disease and that pregnancy is inadvisable. She is put on steroids and her liver biochemistry improves.

◆ **Question 23.10**
What is the long-term prognosis?

Revision

■ Viral hepatitis, pp. 459–461

■ Autoimmune hepatitis, see pp. 468–469

◆ **Answer 23.10**
The liver disease is likely to be controlled with steroids which could be reduced gradually to see if a remission can be sustained. However, there is a significant risk of progression to cirrhosis.

Indigestion

A 55-year-old male accountant attends his doctor's surgery complaining of 'indigestion'. Two years previously the patient had a myocardial infarction from which he made a good recovery. The doctor, suspecting that the patient now has a peptic ulcer, prescribes cimetidine 400 mg twice daily, advises him to stop smoking (the patient smokes approximately 20 cigarettes a day), and asks him to return in 1 month.

◆ Question 24.1
How might cimetidine and the cessation of smoking relieve the patient's symptoms?

Two weeks later the patient vomits blood (haematemesis) and the doctor is called. The patient is pale and sweaty, has a pulse rate of 110/min and his blood pressure is 100/55 mmHg.

◆ Question 24.2
What is the differential diagnosis of the haematemesis?

The doctor calls an ambulance and the patient is admitted to hospital. No further relevant medical history is elicited; in particular, the patient is taking neither aspirin nor an anticoagulant. On examination the patient is noted to have ascites, spider naevi and mild gynaecomastia. The haemoglobin is checked urgently and reported to be 10.5 g/dl. A transfusion of cross-matched group A+ blood is given.

◆ Question 24.3
What is the most likely explanation for the haematemesis?

◆ Question 24.4
What pathological processes are responsible for the ascites, spider naevi and gynaecomastia?

◆ Answer 24.1
Assuming that the 'indigestion' is due to peptic ulceration in the stomach or duodenum, cimetidine reduces gastric acid production by blocking H_2-receptors (class 2 histamine receptors). Smoking is a risk factor for peptic ulceration because it increases gastric acidity; it is logical, therefore, to stop smoking.

'Indigestion' in this age-group probably warrants further investigation because it may be the first manifestation of gastric carcinoma. Cardiac ischaemia may also cause epigastric pain simulating 'indigestion'.

◆ Answer 24.2
Differential diagnosis includes:

- peptic ulcer
- gastric erosions
- gastric carcinoma
- oesophageal varices.

Note also that the patient previously had a myocardial infarction and may, therefore, be taking low-dose aspirin (unlikely to produce gastric erosions at that dose) or an anticoagulant.

◆ Answer 24.3
Ascites, spider naevi and gynaecomastia are together very suggestive of hepatic cirrhosis, complicated in this case by ruptured oesophageal varices due to portal hypertension. (Gynaecomastia may, however, be a side-effect of cimetidine at doses higher than were prescribed in this patient.)

◆ Answer 24.4
Ascites is due to a combination of:

- portal hypertension causing increased pressure in the visceral peritoneal vascular bed (*contd*)

◆ **Question 24.5**

What investigations should be performed?

The results of blood investigations are:

	Patient's values	Normal range
Haemoglobin	13 g/dl (after transfusion)	11.5–5.5 g/dl
Albumin	30 g/l	35–50 g/l
Prothrombin time	1.2 INR[1]	n/a
Alanine aminotransferase (ALT)	60 U/l	5–40 U/l
Aspartate aminotransferase (AST)	80 U/l	5–40 U/l
Bilirubin	15 μmol/l	5–17 μmol/l
Alkaline phosphatase	280 U/l	30–110 U/l
Gamma glutamyl tranferase	65 U/l	0–65 U/l

Upper gastrointestinal endoscopy reveals small oesophageal varices, with no evidence of recent rupture, and an ulcer in the gastric antrum covered with a layer of blood clot; a biopsy is taken from the ulcer.

Four days after admission to hospital, there has been no further haematemesis and the patient is advised to have a percutaneous needle liver biopsy under local anaesthesia.

◆ **Question 24.6**

What should be checked before doing a liver biopsy?

The prothrombin time is 1.2 INR, and hepatitis B and C serology is negative.

A needle liver biopsy is performed under local anaesthesia. A representative appearance is shown in Figure 24.1.

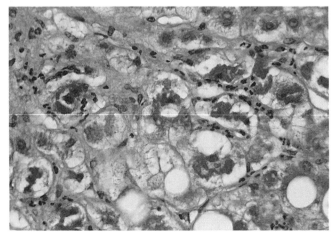

Fig. 24.1

- hypoalbuminaemia causing decreased plasma oncotic pressure (albumin synthesis in the liver may be impaired in cirrhosis)
- secondary aldosteronism, due to failure of the liver to eliminate endogenous aldosterone, causing sodium and water retention.

Spider naevi are due to hyperoestrogenism and are commonly seen during pregnancy. In men they are suggestive of hyperoestrogenism due to liver failure. Gynaecomastia is also due to hyperoestrogenism. Men produce small amounts of hormones with oestrogenic properties, and if the liver fails to metabolise these they can accumulate producing clinical effects.

◆ **Answer 24.5**

- Full blood count and haemoglobin estimation, routine in most cases, but here mandatory because of blood loss
- liver biochemistry — albumin, prothrombin time, transaminases, bilirubin, alkaline phosphatase
- upper gastrointestinal endoscopy
- liver biopsy.

◆ **Answer 24.6**

Mandatory to check the prothrombin time, which may be prolonged in liver disease, due to failure of clotting factor synthesis. Significant prolongation must be corrected. Also wise to check for hepatitis viruses B and C in view of known hazards to medical personnel.

◆ **Question 24.7**
What is the most likely explanation for the liver biopsy appearances?

The patient initially denied excessive alcohol consumption, but now admits to drinking at least 30 units/week. He is advised to stop drinking alcohol.

The gastric biopsy report is received from the histopathology department: 'Fragments of gastric antral type mucosa and granulation tissue, both bearing an acute inflammatory infiltrate. *Helicobacter pylori* are present. There is no evidence of dysplasia or malignancy.'

◆ **Question 24.8**
What is the significance of *H. pylori* in a gastric biopsy?

The patient is treated with tripotassium dicitratobismuthate (with also metronidazole and amoxycillin initially) to eradicate helicobacter. Cimetidine therapy is continued.

◆ **Question 24.9**
What are the long-term complications of the patient's liver condition?

The patient is discharged from hospital, to be followed up as an outpatient. The oesophageal varices are small and there is no evidence that they were the source of haemorrhage.

> **Revision**
>
> ■ Gynaecomastia, see pp. 533–534
>
> ■ Liver biochemistry tests, see 452–455
>
> ■ Alcoholic liver disease, see pp. 462–472
>
> ■ Helicobacter gastritis, see pp. 413–415

◆ **Answer 24.7**
The appearances are strongly suggestive of alcoholic liver injury, a common cause of cirrhosis. Fatty change is seen in many conditions (e.g. alcoholic liver disease, cardiac failure, diabetes mellitus). The intracytoplasmic hyaline material is Mallory's hyalin which, in this context, is consistent with alcoholic liver injury.

◆ **Answer 24.8**
H. pylori is associated with gastritis (type B) and with peptic ulceration, more commonly in the duodenum than the stomach. Eradication of the organism contributes towards ulcer healing and resolution of gastritis and reduces the incidence of relapses. This organism is also associated with gastric lymphoma and, possibly, carcinoma.

◆ **Answer 24.9**
Even if the patient stops drinking alcohol, there is still a high risk of further haematemesis, perhaps fatal, and terminal liver failure. Cirrhosis is also a premalignant condition: liver-cell carcinoma is a well-recognised complication.

[1]International Normalised Ratio (comparing patient's prothrombin time with a control sample).

A chat with a patient

As a general practitioner, you are sent a print-out of all the non-responders to breast screening invitations sent out by your local breast screening unit, for action. Knowing that it is your responsibility to ensure that the maximum number of your patients attend, you send out a personal invitation, to all your patients who have not responded, to see you. A 51-year-old deputy head teacher responds and attends your surgery.

Before you can say anything, she says that her mother developed breast cancer at the age of 55 and despite all the treatment she was given died within 18 months, so she cannot see the point of bothering with screening tests. While listening, you have been thumbing through her notes and you see that she has never attended for cervical smears either.

◆ Question 25.1
What should you explain to her about the general principles of screening tests?

The patient points out that since the death of her mother, she examines her breasts about once per week.

◆ Question 25.2
Isn't this enough?

The patient has heard that they clamp your breasts in a machine for hours and that it is painful.

◆ Question 25.3
Is this correct?

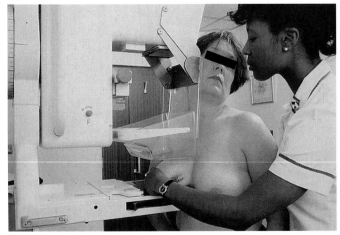

Fig. 25.1

◆ Answer 25.1
Screening is the use of non-invasive tests, which cause little discomfort and are safe, to detect common life-threatening diseases at a stage where their early recognition and treatment reduce morbidity and mortality. Breast cancer kills 15 000 women per year in England and Wales, accounting for 20% of all cancers in women. Early detection improves prognosis and facilitates more conservative surgery in those cases detected.

◆ Answer 25.2
No it is not. Large studies have shown that breast self-examination can detect cancers, but that they are generally over 10 mm diameter when found in this way and have a prognosis no better than average.

◆ Answer 25.3
No. Mammography (Fig. 25.1), which is the basic screening procedure of the United Kingdom Breast Screening Programme takes only a few minutes. It is true that the breasts have to be compressed for good mammograms to be taken, but most patients describe the experience as firm pressure only and only a few experience brief pain.

The patient then asks why, if the screening is so useful, she was not offered it earlier. She remembers reading an article in the *Guardian* saying that the screening programme is a political stunt.

◆ **Question 25.4**
Over what age range are patients offered screening and why?

The patient is afraid that if she attends for screening a quite innocent abnormality might be found and investigated, leading to unnecessary tests or even surgery.

◆ **Question 25.5**
Is there any evidence that she is right?

If the screening tests are so quick and so few people have further investigations, the patient asks, surely the screening is missing cancers.

◆ **Question 25.6**
Is she right?

Finally, the patient asks how the programme can improve survival if a cancer is detected. 'If they find one, it's curtains for you.'

◆ **Question 25.7**
Is she right?

After all your reassurance, the patient agrees to attend for screening. Three weeks later you receive a letter saying that her mammograms were normal and she will be reviewed in 3 years' time.

Revision

■ Breast carcinoma, see pp. 536–550

■ Breast screening, see p. 528

■ Screening, see pp. 69–70

■ Early detection of cancer, see pp. 290–291

◆ **Answer 25.4**
The age range chosen takes into account:

- mammograms are difficult to interpret below age 50 due to density of the breasts
- screening programmes have to be cost-effective; breast cancer becomes commoner with increasing age
- with advanced age, mobility problems make screening very difficult and the number of extra years of life to be gained from screening are reduced.

As a compromise, screening is offered routinely to women over the age of 50.

◆ **Answer 25.5**
Preliminary results show that about 6% of patients are referred for further investigation at an assessment clinic. Thanks to the ability of more detailed diagnostic imaging and fine-needle aspiration cytology to show that many of these patients have innocent impalpable lesions, the biopsy rate is only about 1–3%. Of those biopsied about 2/3 have malignant lesions so overall only less than 1% of women have benign lesions biopsied (each one of which, with hindsight, was an 'unnecessary' procedure).

◆ **Answer 25.6**
The data available so far suggests not. On average 6.2 cancers are being detected per 1000 women screened and this fits in with epidemiological estimates of the prevalence of breast cancer. The expected number of cancers are being found.

◆ **Answer 25.7**
We don't know the effect on survival yet. However on average 1.4 women per 1000 screened are found to have cancers under 10-mm diameter, which have a good prognosis, and screen-detected tumours tend to be better differentiated than those presenting as a mass. An improved prognosis is anticipated.

A pink puffer

A 68-year-old retired lorry driver presents to his general practitioner with a recent increase in breathlessness. The patient says that he has been getting shorter of breath since he retired (at the age of 65 years) and often has to pause for breath when he walks to the local shops. A week ago he developed a cold which he says has 'gone to his chest', and he has a cough with a little green sputum. On further questioning he says that it is unusual for him to have a cough and if he does have one it rarely lasts for more than a month. He has smoked 20 cigarettes a day since he was a teenager.

◆ Question 26.1
Do this patient's symptoms fulfil the definition of chronic bronchitis?

The GP sends the patient to the local hospital for a chest radiograph, which shows hyperinflation with a paucity of vascular markings, and prescribes some antibiotics. He tells the patient to return if his symptoms do not improve and he does not see the patient for 12 months. When the patient comes to the surgery again he complains of a steady increase in breathlessness that is now limiting his daily activities. He can just walk to the corner shop to buy his newspaper and cigarettes but a neighbour has to do his grocery shopping for him. He asks the GP if he can arrange a home help for him because housework makes him too breathless. The patient does not have a cough at the present time. The GP advises him to give up smoking and refers him to a chest physician at the local hospital.

◆ Question 26.2
What possible causes are there for this gradual increase in breathlessness?

On examination at the local hospital the patient has a respiratory rate of 20/min, is thin, breathes through pursed lips and the chest is hyperresonant with loss of the area of cardiac dullness. His respiratory function tests give these results:

Test	Patient's values	Normal range
Vital capacity (VC)	1.81	3.2–4.41
Forced expiratory volume (FEV$_1$)	1.01	1.9–2.91
FEV$_1$/VC ratio	55%	66–78%
Peak expiratory flow rate (PEFR)	200 l/min	460–580 l/min

◆ Answer 26.1
No. Chronic bronchitis is a clinical term defined as chronic cough and sputum for at least 3 months each year for 2 consecutive years.

◆ Answer 26.2
The most likely cause is emphysema. Chronic bronchitis is unlikely to be making a major contribution to the patient's breathlessness since he rarely has a cough or sputum. Pneumoconiosis and diffuse pulmonary fibrosis are other pulmonary causes of slowly progressive breathlessness. Cardiovascular causes would include congestive cardiac failure and recurrent pulmonary embolism. Gross obesity and ankylosing spondylitis are mechanical causes of breathlessness.

and his arterial blood gas results are:

Test	Patient's values	Normal range
Arterial O_2 tension	9.5 KPa	11–13 KPa
Arterial CO_2 tension	5.1 KPa	4.8–6.0 KPa
pH	7.37	7.35–7.45
Standardized HCO_3-	29	24–32

◆ Question 26.3
What pattern of respiratory disease do the respiratory function tests fit into?

◆ Question 26.4
How is the patient maintaining relatively normal arterial O_2 and CO_2 tensions?

Twelve months later the patient is admitted through the accident and emergency with severe breathlessness. On admission his blood gas results are:

Test	Patient's values	Normal range
Arterial O_2 tension	6.5 KPa	11–13 KPa
Arterial CO_2 tension	7.5 KPa	4.8–6.0 KPa
pH	7.21	7.35–7.45
Standardized HCO_3-	31	24–32

◆ Question 26.5
What is likely to have happened now?

◆ Answer 26.3
The patient has reduced vital capacity, a reduced FEV_1/VC ratio and a reduced PEFR. This is an obstructive pattern of disease.

◆ Answer 26.4
The patient is breathing more rapidly than normal and so is able to maintain relatively normal blood gases despite a reduced surface area in the lungs over which gas transfer with the blood may take place.

◆ Answer 26.5
The pulmonary disease which is causing the patient's breathlessness has progressed to a point where an increase in respiratory rate cannot compensate for the lack of surface area for gas exchange. The acidosis without significant renal compensation suggests acute respiratory failure.

The patient dies and a consent autopsy is performed. Figure 26.1 shows the macroscopic appearances of the lungs.

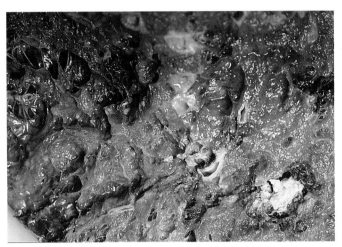

Fig. 26.1

◆ **Question 26.6**
Do these appearances confirm the diagnosis of emphysema?

◆ **Question 26.7**
What is the most likely cause of the emphysema in this case?

◆ **Question 26.8**
What other causes of emphysema are there?

Revision

■ Chronic bronchitis, see pp. 371, 383–384

■ Respiratory function tests, see pp. 365–366

■ Acid-base homeostasis, see pp. 150–152, 356

■ Emphysema, see pp. 384–386

◆ **Answer 26.6**
Yes there are many areas where extensive destruction of lung tissue has produced large holes in the parenchyma (bullae).

◆ **Answer 26.7**
Cigarette smoking.

◆ **Answer 26.8**
Coal-worker's pneumoconiosis (usually a centrilobular pattern), alpha-l-antitrypsin deficiency, local emphysema from fibrotic scarring processes such as old tuberculosis.

Coma!

A 35-year-old man returns to the United Kingdom after 3 weeks travelling through several countries in north Africa in connection with his work. He is a sales representative for a manufacturer of agricultural machinery. He is unmarried and lives alone. Feeling unwell — he thinks he has 'flu' — he telephones his office on Tuesday morning to say that he will not be at work that day. On Wednesday, he still feels unwell so he telephones his general practitioner who advises him to take paracetamol, to rest and to stay off work.

◆ Question 27.1
What is the pathophysiological basis of the symptoms of 'flu'?

By Friday his colleagues are concerned because they have heard nothing further and he is due to be at an agricultural show in France the following week. They telephone him, but there is no reply. One of his colleagues goes to the man's flat, but there is no reply. Two unopened milk bottles are on the doorstep. The police are called and an entry to the flat is effected. The man is lying in bed, apparently asleep, but unrousable.

◆ Question 27.2
What could be responsible for the comatose state?

An ambulance is called and the patient is taken to the nearest hospital. The doctor in the Accident and Emergency department finds no localising neurological signs, and a rapid blood glucose test gives a result at the lower end of the normal range. The ambulance personnel have found nothing in the flat to suggest a drug overdose. The patient's temperature is 40.5°C.

◆ Question 27.3
What is the probable diagnosis?

The patient is admitted to the hospital and a lumbar puncture is performed urgently. A Gram stain of the fluid reveals no organisms.
The doctor in charge of the case telephones the patient's GP to find out if there is any relevant past medical history. The GP checks his records and informs the hospital doctor that he had recently seen the patient before his trip to Africa. He had vaccinated him against typhoid, type C meningococcal meningitis and yellow fever, and issued a prescription for malaria prophylaxis.

◆ Question 27.4
What diagnosis now becomes most likely?

◆ Answer 27.1
'Flu' is the layman's generic name for any illness characterised by pyrexia, malaise, muscular aches and symptoms of an upper respiratory tract infection. Not all cases are due to influenza virus. Irrespective of the specific cause, the signs and symptoms are almost entirely due to interleukins (peptides produced by leucocytes) acting on the central nervous system (i.e. on the thermoregulatory centre in the hypothalamus).

◆ Answer 27.2
Coma has many causes including:

- cerebrovascular accident ('stroke')
- meningitis
- hypoglycaemia
- diabetic ketoacidosis
- drug overdose
- malaria.

◆ Answer 27.3
The findings seem to exclude diabetic causes (hypoglycaemia due to insulin therapy, or ketoacidosis), cerebrovascular accident and drug overdose. The possibility of an infectious cause must be considered seriously and this is favoured by the high temperature.

◆ Answer 27.4
Malaria. Coma is a feature of cerebral malaria. Patients often forget to take their malaria prophylaxis and even when taken it does not offer complete protection.

◆ **Question 27.5**
How would you investigate the possibility of malaria?

A blood film has the appearance shown in Figure 27.1.

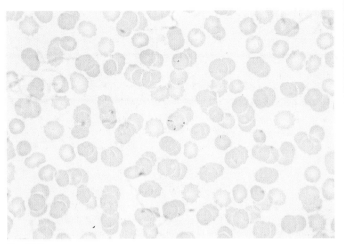

Fig. 27.1

◆ **Question 27.6**
What does this blood film show?

Malaria is diagnosed and treatment with quinine is instituted. Over the next few days the patient's temperature falls to normal and he gradually recovers consciousness. One week after admission to hospital he is able to walk around the ward and 10 days after admission he is discharged.

Revision

■ Malaria, see pp. 90, 671, 853

■ Interleukins, see p. 203

◆ **Answer 27.5**
The best way of making a firm diagnosis is to look for the malaria parasite in the blood. This is usually done by examining a thick blood film.

◆ **Answer 27.6**
Malaria parasites (plasmodia) in red cells.

Chest pain

A 64-year-old retired teacher is walking around a marquee at a flower show when she experiences a pain in her chest. The pain is central with some radiation down her left arm. She sits down by some fuschias and the pain lessens in intensity after 5 minutes rest but persists. A stall holder asks her if she is all right; she says that she sometimes gets chest pain on walking 400 metres or more but that the pain always disappears when she rests or when she uses the spray which her general practitioner prescribed for her.

◆ **Question 28.1**
What pathologies may cause chest pain?

◆ **Question 28.2**
What cause is most likely in this case given the description of the symptoms and the patient's history, and why are the other causes less likely?

Since the chest pain has not completely gone the stall holder calls an ambulance and the lady is taken to the local hospital where she is seen by the senior house officer in the Accident and Emergency department. The doctor takes a history, performs a clinical examination and then orders some tests.

◆ **Question 28.3**
What tests would be most relevant to the diagnosis and management of this patient's disease?

The ECG showed elevation of the ST segments in the lateral chest leads. No significant increase in the depth of the Q waves were identified.
The results of the cardiac related enzymes are:

Enzyme	Patient's values	Normal range
Creatine phosphokinase	123 U/l	Female 24–170 U/l
Lactate dehydrogenase	121 U/l	100–265 U/l

◆ **Answer 28.1**
Ischaemic heart disease (angina pectoris, myocardial infarction), pericarditis, aortic aneurysm, pulmonary embolism and infarction, pneumothorax, gastro-oesophageal reflux, neural pathology (herpes zoster, compression of nerve roots due to degenerative processes in the cervical spine).

◆ **Answer 28.2**
Ischaemic heart disease is the most likely pathology given the association with exercise and the site of the pain (with radiation down the left arm). Pericarditis may produce a pain which is more intense on inspiration and would not be associated with exercise. The pain produced by gastro-oesophageal reflux is usually worsened by lying supine and may be related to eating. Aortic aneurysms and pulmonary embolism/infarction would tend to produce pain with a sudden onset but which would then remain constant or worsen; pulmonary embolism/infarction is often associated with breathlessness. Pneumothorax would produce a pain that was related to respiratory movements. Neural causes would tend to produce a constant pain.

◆ **Answer 28.3**
An electrocardiogram (ECG) and measurement of cardiac-related enzymes could confirm the presence of ischaemic heart disease and suggest what type of ischaemic process is present.

◆ **Question 28.4**
Is this patient likely to have had a myocardial infarction?

Since this patient does not appear to have had a myocardial infarction then her symptoms (increased pain which is not completely relieved by rest) puts her into the category of unstable angina. Figure 28.1 is a diagram of an atheromatous plaque such as may be found in a coronary artery:

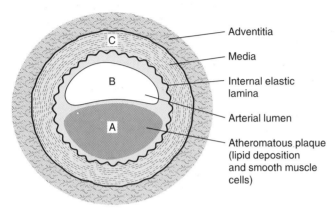

Adventitia

Media

Internal elastic lamina

Arterial lumen

Atheromatous plaque (lipid deposition and smooth muscle cells)

Fig. 28.1

◆ **Question 28.5**
What types of pathological processes could occur at the different sites (A–C) marked on the diagram which could cause decrease in the luminal area and so precipitate unstable or increased angina?

◆ **Question 28.6**
What therapeutic measures could be used to combat these pathological processes?

Revision

■ Ischaemic heart disease, see pp. 335–339

■ Atheroma, see pp. 310–316

■ Thrombosis, see pp. 166–169

■ Infarction, see pp. 114, 173–178

◆ **Answer 28.4**
There is no evidence from the cardiac-related enzymes that the patient has had a myocardial infarction but it can take a few hours for these to rise after a myocardial infarction; it takes time for the membranes of the necrotic myocardial cells to breakdown to allow enzyme release. Further measurement of enzymes would be required to exclude a myocardial infarction completely.

◆ **Answer 28.5**
At site 'A' haemorrhage into the atheromatous plaque could cause an increase in the size of the plaque and thus narrowing of the luminal area. At site 'B' thrombus could form on the luminal surface of the plaque causing increased narrowing and reduction of blood flow; if thrombus completely filled the lumen a myocardial infarction would occur unless collateral vessels were very plentiful; partial occlusion could produce unstable angina. It is possible that contraction of smooth muscle in the media at 'C' could cause further narrowing of the luminal area; contraction of muscle beneath the plaque is unlikely to cause narrowing because the plaque itself would resist compression.

◆ **Answer 28.6**
Aspirin (in low doses) inhibits platelet aggregation which initiates thrombus formation on the luminal surface of the plaque. Thrombolytic agents, such as streptokinase, can lyse intraluminal thrombi. Glyceryl trinitrate, which would have been present in the spray prescribed by the patient's general practitioner, causes smooth-muscle relaxation and may relieve vascular spasm in coronary arteries.

A numb foot

A 30-year-old man with no relevant past medical history develops lower lumbar back pain.

◆ Question 29.1
What are the causes of back pain?

The patient does not seek medical attention and relieves the pain with paracetamol. The pain recurs for several weeks approximately every year for the next 10 years. During one particularly severe episode, he is referred by his general practitioner to an orthopaedic surgeon. A radiograph of the spine shows no abnormality, but physical examination reveals marked limitation of straight-leg raising on the right side.

◆ Question 29.2
What is the most likely diagnosis?

Neurological examination reveals loss of the ankle reflex on the right side.

◆ Question 29.3
What nerve root is most likely to be compressed?

The patient is advised to wear a plastic corset for the next 3 months and to take mild analgesia. Three months later the patient is reassessed: the pain is much less and the straight-leg raising has improved. The patient is discharged.

Ten years after the last episode of severe pain there is a further recurrence. This is associated with paraesthesia in the lateral aspect of the right foot and marked scoliosis.

◆ Question 29.4
What is the significance of the paraesthesiae and scoliosis?

The patient is referred to a neurologist. Clinical examination reveals sensory impairment to light touch on the lateral aspect of the right foot and lower leg. There is no apparent muscle weakness or wasting. There is a marked scoliosis of the lower thoracic and the lumbar spine. The patient is referred for a magnetic resonance imaging (MRI) scan.

◆ Answer 29.1
Back pain is common and can be either referred from internal organs (e.g. pancreatitis may cause upper lumbar pain, dysmenorrhoea may be associated with lower lumbar pain) or due to local problems. Local causes of lower lumbar back pain include:

- minor strain or injury
- degenerative disc disease
- osteopenic vertebral collapse
- infections within and around the spine
- arthopathies affecting spinal joints
- tumours, primary (e.g. myeloma) or secondary (e.g. metastatic carcinoma).

◆ Answer 29.2
The relatively long history virtually excludes neoplasia. The normal spinal radiograph and the absence of apparent disease in other body systems virtually excludes inflammatory conditions such as infections or arthropathies. However, the limited straight-leg raising is an important diagnostic test indicating nerve root compression, probably by a herniation of degenerate nucleus pulposus from an intervertebral disc.

◆ Answer 29.3
The L5/S1 nerve root, the commonest level to be compressed by degenerative disc disease.

◆ Answer 29.4
Paraesthesiae may be an indication of sensory nerve root compression. Muscle weakness may be a manifestation of motor nerve root compression. The scoliosis is due to reflex muscular spasm.

◆ **Question 29.5**
What is the justification for an MRI scan when the patient is already diagnosed as having degenerative disc disease?

The one image from the MRI scan is shown in Figure 29.1.

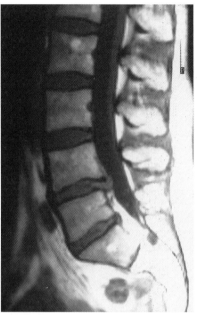

Fig. 29.1   Courtesy of Dr T Powell, Sheffield

◆ **Question 29.6**
What pathological abnormality is revealed by the MRI scan?

The patient is advised that the prolapse will not resolve by conservative management (e.g. bed rest and analgesia) and that its size and location threatens other neurological functions. The prolapsed disc material is, therefore, removed surgically and, with physiotherapy, the patient makes an excellent recovery.

Revision

■ Degenerative intervertebral disc disease, see p. 813

■ Neural and spinal compression, see pp. 838–839

◆ **Answer 29.5**
Degenerative disc disease is very common. Any new symptoms could be due to the development of a new disease. Furthermore, an MRI scan enables precise assessment of the location and size of the prolapsed or sequestrated degenerative disc material.

◆ **Answer 29.6**
The MRI scan reveals a large prolapse of the L5/S1 disc resulting in nerve root compression.

Postmenopausal bleeding

A 68-year-old woman goes to see her general practitioner complaining of vaginal blood loss. The GP takes a history and finds that the woman had the menopause around the age of 48 years and until the last 2 months had had no vaginal blood loss or discharge. The GP performs a vaginal examination and finds that the cervix has a smooth surface and there appears to be a small amount of blood coming from the external os. The GP then takes a smear from the cervix and refers the patient to the local gynaecologist.

◆ **Question 30.1**
What is the most likely source of the bleeding?

◆ **Question 30.2**
If the source is endometrial what is the most likely pathology?

The gynaecologist takes an endometrial biopsy, using a Pipelle sampler, in the outpatient department and sends the specimen for histopathological examination. Figure 30.1 is a microscopic picture of normal endometrium, and Figure 30.2 is a microscopic picture of the patient's endometrium.

◆ **Answer 30.1**
The endometrium, but other sources should be sought at vaginal examination such as the cervix or the vagina.

◆ **Answer 30.2**
Carcinoma of the endometrium.

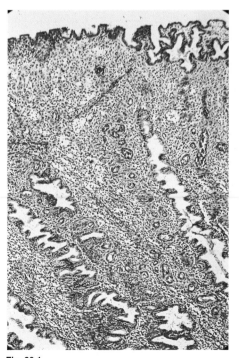
Fig. 30.1

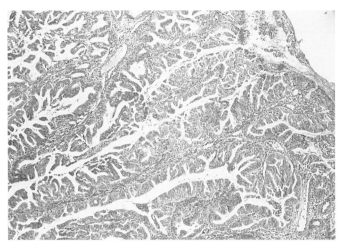

Fig. 30.2

◆ Question 30.3
What differences can you see between the two pictures?

After seeing the histopathological report on the Pipelle specimen the gynaecologist arranges for the patient to be admitted for a hysterectomy. The hysterectomy specimen is sent to the histopathology laboratory and has the macroscopic appearances shown in Figure 30.3.

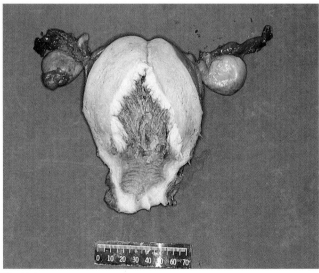

Fig. 30.3

◆ Question 30.4
What features will the histopathologist assess?

◆ Answer 30.3
There is a much higher ratio of gland epithelium to stroma in the patient's biopsy than in the normal endometrium. The gland epithelium has an abnormal architecture with 'back to back' glands. Examination at a higher magnification would show the nuclei of the epithelial cells in the patient's biopsy to be pleomorphic and hyperchromatic. The appearances are those of endometrial adenocarcinoma.

◆ Answer 30.4
The histopathologist will examine blocks from the tumour to confirm the histological type of tumour and to grade the tumour. Blocks will be taken from the myometrium beneath the tumour to assess the extent of tumour invasion. The ovaries, fallopian tubes and cervix will also be sampled to look for any related or incidental pathology.

◆ **Question 30.5**

What is the most important prognostic factor in endometrial adenocarcinoma?

◆ **Question 30.6**

What associated pathology could be present in the ovaries (which was absent in this case)?

Revision

■ Endometrial adenocarcinoma, see pp. 565–566

■ Ovarian neoplasms, see pp. 570–576

◆ **Answer 30.5**

The extent of myometrial invasion at the time of diagnosis is the most important prognostic factor.

◆ **Answer 30.6**

Sometimes granulosa cell tumours may be found in the ovaries of women with endometrial adenocarcinoma. These tumours are derived from the sex-cord stromal cells and convert hormonal precursors to oestrogens; they may therefore produce excess oestrogens and this hormonal environment is associated with endometrial hyperplasia and endometrial adenocarcinoma.

'He's just not himself anymore'

A 45-year-old school teacher is just not himself anymore. Apart from a depressive illness when he was a student, he has had no serious medical problems. He is married — his wife is a part-time laboratory technician — with two children, both sons, aged 18 and 15.

He is finding it increasingly difficult to cope with his work. The pupils at the school seem more disruptive than ever. Last week, during a geography lesson, he had to dismiss the class early because he 'lost his concentration'. Fortunately, the headteacher was approachable and understanding and suggested that he should take some time off work.

◆ Question 31.1
To what extent, if any, could this situation be attributed to illness?

Unfortunately, this situation worsens. Over the next few weeks his wife notices that he is forgetful and withdrawn. Together they see their general practitioner who diagnoses a depressive illness and prescribes an antidepressant. There is no improvement over the next few months.

◆ Question 31.2
What is the pathophysiological basis of depressive illness?

One afternoon, the police are called to a clothes shop because the patient is suspected of 'shoplifting'. The police notice that his speech is slurred. He is also unable to remember where he lives. The police suspect he is ill rather than intoxicated, and this is confirmed by the police surgeon. The police decide to release him without charge, and they drive him home, his wife having reported his unexpected absence to the police. The police surgeon writes a report to the man's general practitioner; this prompts the GP to make a home visit. He refers the patient to the local psychiatrist.

The psychiatrist finds no evidence of a depressive illness. The most likely explanation for the man's behaviour is considered to be a neurodegenerative disorder or a space-occupying lesion.

◆ Question 31.3
What is a neurodegenerative disorder?

◆ Answer 31.1
The most likely explanation is that he is suffering from stress due to what he perceives as the increasingly disruptive pupils. However, people who are ill from any cause (or even healthy!) may find ordinary life stressful.

◆ Answer 31.2
Irrespective of whether the depressive illness is classified as 'reactive' (i.e. triggered by adverse life events) or 'endogenous', there is a reduction in catecholamine concentrations in post-synaptic nerve endings.

◆ Answer 31.3
Neurodegenerative disorders are conditions causing dementia or impaired cognition and mentation. They include:

- Creutzfeldt — Jakob disease
- cerebral atherosclerosis
- Alzheimer's disease
- senile dementia.

◆ **Question 31.4**
What is a space-occupying lesion?

The patient is referred to a neurologist. Investigations fail to reveal any localised lesion. The most likely diagnosis is considered to be a neurodegenerative disorder, probably Alzheimer's disease.

◆ **Question 31.5**
What is Alzheimer's disease?

◆ **Question 31.6**
What is the cause of Alzheimer's disease?

The patient's condition progressively worsens over the next year, by which time he unable to dress, shave, wash or feed himself. He is cared for at home by his wife with nursing support. Eventually his condition is so poor that his family cannot cope and he is admitted to a local hospice.

While there he falls out of bed, causing a fractured humerus. He then develops bronchopneumonia and dies a week later. Because of the recent injury, which may have accelerated his death, the coroner is informed and a medicolegal autopsy is performed.

◆ **Question 31.7**
What autopsy findings would support the diagnosis of Alzheimer's disease?

Three months after the patient's death, his son visits the family's GP to ask about whether there is any chance that his father's disease could be inherited and, therefore, passed down the family from father to son.

◆ **Question 31.8**
How is the risk of Alzheimer's disease inherited?

Revision

■ Alzheimer's disease, see pp. 864–865

◆ **Answer 31.4**
In the context of the central nervous system (CNS), a space-occupying lesion is a localised swelling, such as a tumour, compressing adjacent structures and possibly causing raised intracranial pressure.

◆ **Answer 31.5**
Alzheimer's disease is the commonest cause of pre-senile dementia. Its salient features are indistinguishable from senile dementia, the principal distinction being its occurrence at a younger age.

◆ **Answer 31.6**
The cause is unknown. However, genetic and environmental causes have been postulated. There is certainly a genetic component in families with a higher than expected incidence of the disease. Dietary aluminium has also been incriminated, but the evidence is weak and controversial.

◆ **Answer 31.7**
The changes resemble those seen in natural ageing. The brain is small, often less than 1000 g, with cortical atrophy most marked in the temporal and frontal regions. Histologically, there will be two abnormalities:

• senile plaques (extracellular) with amyloid in their cores
• neurofibrillary tangles (intracellular).

◆ **Answer 31.8**
Most cases of Alzheimer's disease are sporadic. However, in families with a higher than expected incidence, the condition is inherited as an autosomal dominant trait. Current evidence favours an abnormality on chromosome 21. Similar CNS changes are seen in Down's syndrome which is frequently associated with trisomy 21.

A specific tumour marker

A 32-year-old woman has a positive pregnancy test and attends antenatal clinic. By her dates she should be 8 weeks pregnant. She is well except for nausea and morning vomitting which she says is worse than during her previous pregnancy 2 years earlier. A routine ultrasound scan shows no evidence of a fetal pole and there are multiple echogenic lucencies. An evacuation of the contents of the uterus is performed under general anaesthesia.

Figure 32.1 shows histological sections of material from a normal early pregnancy: Figure 32.2 shows the histological appearance of material removed from this patient's uterus.

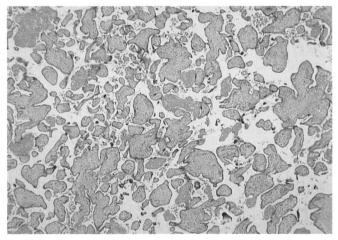

Fig. 32.1

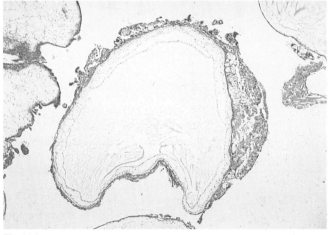

Fig. 32.2

◆ **Question 32.1**
What differences can you see between the two pictures?

◆ **Answer 32.1**
The chorionic villi in the material from the patient are much larger and have empty cystic central areas (cisternae). The trophoblastic tissue around the edge of the villi is hyperplastic. These histological appearances (and the absence of fetal tissue) are of a complete hydatidiform mole.

◆ **Question 32.2**
What complications can arise after a complete
hydatidiform mole?

◆ **Question 32.3**
How should this patient be followed up?

Figure 32.3 is a graph of the patient's urinary HCG levels in
the 6 months following evacuation of the uterine contents:

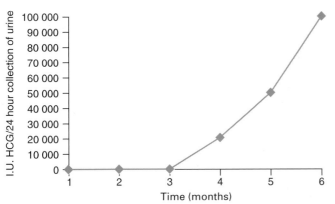

Fig. 32.3

◆ **Question 32.4**
What is the cause of these results?

The gynaecologist removes the patient's uterus which has the
macroscopic appearances shown in Figure 32.4. This shows
that the fundic part of the uterus contains tissue which still
has cystic structures within it. Microscopic examination
shows that chorionic villi are present within the myometrium
and myometrial vessels. The appearances in this specimen
are of invasive hydatidiform mole.

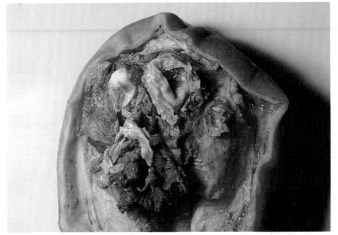

Fig. 32.4

◆ **Answer 32.2**
In a small number of cases there may be
persistent trophoblastic disease where
the trophoblast remains in the uterus
and may undergo malignant change.

◆ **Answer 32.3**
Trophoblast produces human chorionic
gonadotrophin (HCG) which is not
normally found in the non-pregnant
state. The patient should be advised to
avoid pregnancy and serum and urine
levels of HCG should be measured.

◆ **Answer 32.4**
Persistent trophoblastic disease.

◆ **Question 32.5**
What is the main complication of this condition?

◆ **Answer 32.5**
Uterine perforation.

◆ **Question 32.6**
What other forms of persistent trophoblastic disease are there?

◆ **Answer 32.6**
Exaggerated placental site reaction and, most importantly, choriocarcinoma. Choriocarcinoma is a malignant neoplasm of the trophoblast which commonly metastasises but is very sensitive to treatment with chemotherapy.

HCG is a very specific tumour marker and, as this case illustrates, is useful in detecting persistent trophoblastic disease. An ideal tumour marker would be absent in healthy individuals so any detectable levels would be indicative of disease, it would also be specific for a particular sort of tumour. In reality most tumour markers do not have these ideal properties but there are a few which are useful in the detection and management of human tumours.

◆ **Question 32.7**
What other tumour markers can you name and which tumours do they relate to?

◆ **Answer 32.7**
Alpha-fetoprotein is often raised in liver cell carcinoma, peptide hormones (such as insulin and gastrin) will have raised levels in tumours of the cells which produce them (APUDomas), vanillyl mandelic acid (a metabolite of catecholamines) may be detected in the urine of subjects with phaeochromocytoma, carcinoembryonic antigen may be raised in cases of gastrointestinal adenocarcinoma but it is not very specific.

Revision

■ Pathology of pregnancy, see pp. 576–584

■ Placental tumours, see pp. 576–577

■ Tumour markers, see pp. 260, 612–613

'They're talking about me'

A 23-year-old unemployed man is arrested by the police for 'shoplifting' in a supermarket. While being arrested, he punches one of the police officers and renders him unconscious. (The policeman recovers consciousness within a few minutes, but is taken to hospital and admitted overnight for observation; the following day he is discharged home.)

The police recognise the man as a well-known intravenous drug abuser. The man's appearance is rather dishevelled, his behaviour is bizarre and, when being interviewed at the police station, he is unable to give a coherent account of himself. He seems to be 'talking to himself' rather than to the police officers. He is not drunk. The police are worried about him and call the police surgeon. The young man tells the doctor that he was stealing from the shop because 'God told him to'. The police are unconvinced by this explanation and want to charge the man with grievous bodily harm. The doctor, however, provisionally diagnoses schizophrenia.

◆ Question 33.1
What features support the diagnosis of schizophrenia?

The doctor advises the police that the man, having already punched a police officer, may be a risk to the public and that he may require urgent psychiatric attention. Under current mental health legislation, the man is taken to a secure unit at a local psychiatric hospital. After observation, the man's behaviour is considered consistent with the diagnosis of schizophrenia. He is treated with chlorpromazine.

Two weeks later, the nursing staff notice that their patient is jaundiced.

◆ Question 33.2
What are the more likely explanations for the development of jaundice in this case?

◆ Answer 33.1
The diagnosis of schizophrenia could not be made with certainty under these circumstances. The man could be feigning mental illness to escape arrest. Nevertheless, the doctor's first duty is to his patient and he is wise to consider the possibility very seriously.

◆ Answer 33.2
The patient is an intravenous drug abuser and may, therefore, have hepatitis B or C virus infection. Alternatively, the jaundice could be an adverse reaction to chlorpromazine.

Blood samples are taken for liver biochemistry and for testing for evidence of human immunodeficiency virus (HIV), hepatitis B and C infection. The biochemistry shows:

	Patient's values	Normal range
Bilirubin	28 μmol/l	5–17 μmol/l
Alanine aminotransferase (ALT)	45 U/l	5–40 U/l
Alkaline phosphatase	45 U/l	30–110 U/l

The patient is positive for hepatitis B (HBsAg) and hepatitis C (anti-HCV), but HIV negative. The local hepatologist is asked to see the patient. A liver biopsy is performed (Fig. 33.1).

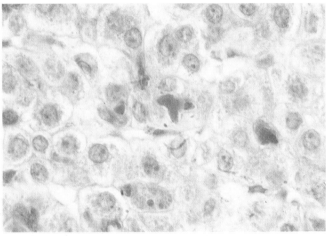

Fig. 33.1

◆ Question 33.3
What is the main abnormality in this liver biopsy and how does it help to resolve the differential diagnosis?

The patient's treatment is changed from chlorpromazine to haloperidol. Within a week the jaundice has started to fade and it clears within a month. By this time the patient's psychiatric condition has much improved. The police don't consider it worth pursuing charges, even for assault, in view of the man's mental state at the time of committing the offences. The man is discharged into the care of a local hostel for drug addicts.

Six months after the original episode, the man is found unconscious in his room at the hostel. An ambulance is called and he is taken to hospital.

◆ Question 33.4
What is the most likely explanation for his condition?

◆ Answer 33.3
The main abnormality is intrahepatic cholestasis: there are threads and plugs of bile lying between the hepatocytes; the hepatocytes are virtually normal and there is little inflammatory reaction. This favours jaundice due to chlorpromazine rather than viral hepatitis; the latter would be associated with more evidence of liver cell injury.

◆ Answer 33.4
Bearing in mind the circumstances (drug abuse, schizophrenia), drug overdose should be strongly suspected. Other possibilities include head injury (of which there is no sign), spontaneous intracranial haemorrhage (such as subarachnoid haemorrhage), and diabetic or hypoglycaemic coma (he is not diabetic).

The ambulance staff found an empty paracetamol bottle near the patient. A blood sample is taken for urgent paracetamol assay and the patient has a stomach washout. The patient is admitted to the hospital. The plasma paracetamol level is 220 mg/l, confirming the suspected overdose and at a level sufficient to warrant antidote treatment (assuming that about 8 hours had elapsed since taking the overdose). The patient is given acetylcysteine.

◆ Question 33.5
What is the rationale of giving acetylcysteine?

During the next few days the patient's condition deteriorates. He becomes jaundiced and starts bleeding from venepuncture sites. He remains unconscious. His urine output falls. One week after admission he dies in liver failure.

◆ Question 33.6
What would you write on the death certificate?

The coroner directs an autopsy to be performed.

◆ Question 33.7
How should the pathologist prepare for this case?

The pathologist confirms that death was due to liver failure. The liver weighs 900 g.

◆ Question 33.8
What would you expect the liver to show histologically?

Revision

- Jaundice, see pp. 456–457
- Iatrogenic disease, see pp. 25–26
- Liver biopsy, see p. 455
- Autopsy, see pp. 75–76

◆ Answer 33.5
Paracetamol is metabolised in the liver where, if the levels are toxic, the metabolites bind to the lipid membranes of cells. Acetylcysteine is a glutathione precursor and protects the liver from the toxic effects of paracetamol metabolites.

◆ Answer 33.6
The patient's death is not from natural causes. In most modern legislative systems, the case should be referred to the appropriate legal officer (for example, the coroner in England and Wales, or the procurator fiscal in Scotland). The patient's doctor is not empowered to issue death certificates in cases where death is known or suspected to be due to unnatural causes.

◆ Answer 33.7
The pathologist should ensure that the post-mortem room was suitable for dealing with known or suspected high-risk cases (HBV and HCV are category 3 pathogens).

◆ Answer 33.8
Coagulative centrilobular necrosis. This pattern of necrosis is typical of paracetamol toxicity.

Heartburn

A 48-year-old taxi driver has been troubled by 'heartburn' for several years. When questioned by his general practitioner, he says that he feels a burning sensation in his chest, worse on lying down, particularly after eating a meal. He is worried that it could be 'heart disease'. He smokes about 20 cigarettes a day and drinks about 10 pints of beer. He is overweight.

◆ **Question 34.1**
What is the most likely explanation for 'heartburn'?

◆ **Question 34.2**
What factors contribute to gastro-oesophageal reflux?

The patient is advised to reduce weight, stop smoking and cut down on his drinking. He is also told to buy some antacid tablets and suck them whenever he feels the burning pain.

The patient returns 3 months later, still complaining of heartburn. He is referred to the gastroenterologist at his local hospital.

The gastroenterologist finds nothing abnormal on routine clinical examination, other than that the patient is still over-weight. The patient is told he should have an endoscopic examination of the oesophagus to investigate the condition.

At endoscopy the upper two-thirds of the oesophagus are normal, but the mucosa of the lower third appears red and ulcerated. A biopsy is taken 300 mm from the incisors (Fig. 34.1).

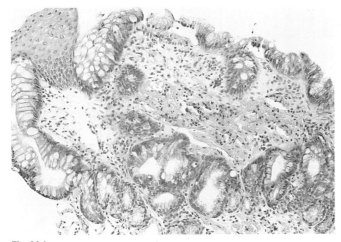

Fig. 34.1

◆ **Answer 34.1**
The word 'heartburn' (pyrosis) is not very specific in terms of diagnostic associations, but most probably he has reflux oesophagitis. Acidic gastric contents pass into the lower oesophagus and irritate, inflame and sometimes ulcerate the mucosa.

◆ **Answer 34.2**
In many cases no underlying cause is detected. However, reflux may be due to:

- hiatus hernia
- obesity
- pregnancy.

◆ Question 34.3
How would you interpret these histological appearances?

The patient returns to the clinic 10 days later. The histology report on the oesophageal biopsy reads: 'Three fragments of glandular mucosa bearing an acute inflammatory infiltrate. The epithelial cells show nuclear enlargement and increased mitotic activity.'

The patient is prescribed a stronger antacid. He returns 3 months later and feels much better. His heartburn has almost gone. He is told that he should return in 1 year for a further endoscopy.

The patient's taxi firm runs into financial difficulties and he is made redundant. He fails to attend for repeat endoscopy. After being unemployed for a year, he and his family leave their home town and move elsewhere. Ten years after first presenting with 'heartburn', his symptoms return. He has lost 1 stone in weight during the last 3 months and now has difficulty in swallowing.

◆ Question 34.4
What is the differential diagnosis of difficulty in swallowing (dysphagia)?

He is referred to the local hospital. He is found to be anaemic. A firm lymph node is palpable in the left supraclavicular fossa; it is biopsied and sent for a histological opinion (Fig. 34.2).

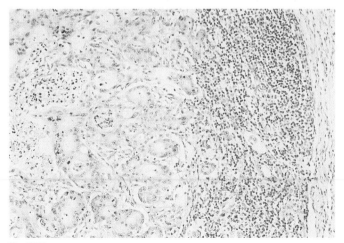

Fig. 34.2

◆ Question 34.5
What could explain the histological features of this lymph node?

◆ Answer 34.3
First, the presence of glandular mucosa at 300 mm is abnormal and indicates metaplasia. The nuclear enlargement and mitotic activity is probably a regenerative response to inflammatory injury.

◆ Answer 34.4

- benign oesophageal stricture
- oesophageal carcinoma
- achalasia of the cardia
- hysteria
- oesophageal or pharyngeal pouch.

◆ Answer 34.5
The lymph node contains neoplastic glandular epithelium; this is metastatic adenocarcinoma. Adenocarcinoma in a supraclavicular lymph node is most likely to have come from the upper gastrointestinal tract.

Oesophagoscopy reveals an ulcerated lesion in the lower third, partly occluding the lumen. It is biopsied and adeno-carcinoma is confirmed.

◆ Question 34.6
Is there any relationship between the previous oesophageal pathology and the carcinoma?

The patient and his family are told the diagnosis and also that, because the tumour has already spread, there is no point in subjecting the patient to the risks associated with oesophagectomy. A tube will be inserted in the lower oesoph-agus to allow liquid and semisolid food to reach the stomach. The patient survives 3 months.

At autopsy, widespread metastatic adenocarcinoma is found with deposits in numerous lymph nodes and in the liver.

Revision

- Metaplasia, see pp. 107–108
- Barrett's oesophagus, see pp. 409–410
- Oesophageal carcinoma, see p. 410
- Preneoplastic lesions, see p. 273

◆ Answer 34.6
The glandular metaplasia (Barrett's oesophagus) predisposes to adenocarcinoma of the lower oesophagus. It is a premalignant condition.

Left shift

A 35-year-old woman presents in Accident and Emergency having cut her finger on a can opener the day before and it is still actively bleeding. On examination it is a minor cut not requiring sutures. There is no sensory or motor deficit and there is no vascular deficit distal to the wound. The patient is one of heterozygous twins, has no significant medical history and the general examination is within normal limits. Direct questioning reveals no personal or family history of note and there is no history of excessive bleeding or bruising. She is given a tetanus booster as she last had one in school and the wound is cleaned and dressed.

◆ **Question 35.1**
What test would you do?

Her white cell count is $50 \times 10^9/l$. She is referred to the medical firm who perform a battery of tests.

◆ **Question 35.2**
How would you investigate this patient further?

When the diagnosis is established a course of treatment is begun.

◆ **Question 35.3**
How would you treat this patient?

◆ **Answer 35.1**
Some form of clotting test is needed. Since clotting is such a complex system involving vascular integrity, thrombocytes and the clotting cascade, a screening test that is non-specific is the most economic investigation. In practice these are currently measured individually. This patient's results showed a relative thrombocytopenia and a 'left shift' which indicates a relative increase in white cell numbers. An increase in white cells can occur for a number of reasons including reaction to infection and neoplastic proliferation of white cell as well as increases seen as general effects of systemic disease.

◆ **Answer 35.2**
On the wards it was found that the increased numbers of white cells were myeloid cells, many of them abnormal (Figs 35.1 & 35.2), there was a mild normocytic, normochromic anaemia and marked thrombocytopenia. The clotting cascade and the capillaries were normal. Bone marrow trephine showed increased cellularity with 80% blast cells.

◆ **Answer 35.3**
Start her on a course of combination chemotherapy together with prophylactic antibiotics.

She has a stormy course on treatment with numerous infections and no significant remission.

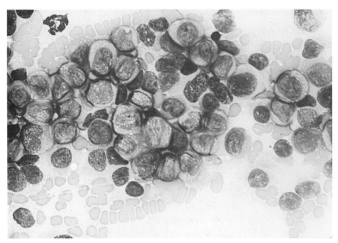

Fig. 35.1

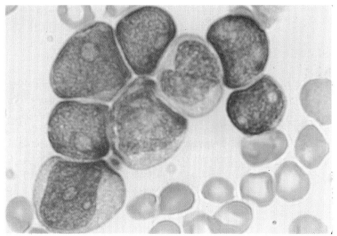

Fig. 35.2

◆ Question 35.4
Are there any other lines of treatment?

Within several days of this treatment she develops a skin rash and acute systemic fever and malaise. No evidence of infection can be found. A skin biopsy is taken.

◆ Question 35.5
What might the skin biopsy show?

◆ Question 35.6
Is GVHD a common complication of heart or renal transplants?

◆ Answer 35.4
Since she had a twin who was willing to donate marrow, a bone marrow transplant was performed. In this treatment the patient's own bone marrow is wiped out in order to destroy the malignant cells. A transplant of closely matched donor marrow is then introduced with the hope that these cells will repopulate the patient's marrow.

◆ Answer 35.5
The skin biopsy showed a lichenoid reaction typical of severe graft-versus-host disease (GVHD). This occurs when the bone marrow transplant is not an exact transplant antigen match with the recipient. In this patient's case the donor marrow came from a heterozygous twin and the match was very close but not identical; a homozygous twin would have had an exact match. GVHD occurs under these circumstances of mismatch because the transplanted white cells recognize the host major histocompatability complexes on the cell surfaces as different to their own and they attempt to destroy them. This can result in destruction of tissues in most organs of the body.

Rarely, deposits of malignant myeloid cells can occur in the skin. These are often green in colour due to the large amounts of myeloperoxidase that they may contain and for this reason they are known as chloromas.

◆ Answer 35.6
No. GVHD is caused by the introduction of alien lymphoid cells into a patient, these cells then see the patient as foreign and attempt to reject him or her. In heart and renal transplants there is no significant introduction of immunocompetent cells into the host and so there is generally no problem of GVHD, although the host may attempt to reject the graft.

In spite of active treatment she develops a series of infections and mucosal bleeding and dies within 3 months of diagnosis.

◆ **Question 35.7**
What will the autopsy show?

Revision

■ Coagulation cascade, see pp. 733–742

■ Haematological investigations, see pp. 7, 70, 683–698

■ Transplantation immunology, see p. 211

■ Graft-versus-host disease, see pp. 211, 476

■ Opportunistic infections, see p. 216

◆ **Answer 35.7**
The clinicians who deal with these patients attempt to get autopsies on all leukaemic patients who die in this particular hospital in order to evaluate the disease and their treatment of it. At autopsy the patient had evidence of GVHD in numerous organs including skin, muscle, heart, gut and brain and this was confirmed histologically. There was spontaneous bleeding in many organs and there was a subphrenic abscess. The lungs showed infection with both bacteria and fungi but there was no acute inflammatory infiltrate due to the marked suppression of all white cells.

A failure of screening

A 55-year-old woman who works in a food processing plant goes to see her general practitioner complaining of a persistent vaginal discharge. Her GP enquires about her past reproductive and gynaecological history and finds that she has four children, the first of which she had when she was 17 years old. In her mid-30s she had a cervical dilation and endometrial curettage when she complained of heavy periods but no abnormality was found and she became menopausal around the age of 50 years. She had had a cervical smear taken at the time of endometrial curettage but had had no subsequent smears. She says that the vaginal discharge does not have an offensive smell, is slightly blood-stained and is not like 'thrush' which she has had in the past. The general practitioner, with the assistance of the practice nurse, takes a high vaginal swab which is sent for microbiological culture and a cervical smear which is sent for cytological examination.

Under the microscope, in the pathology laboratory of the local hospital, the pathologist finds the cells shown in Figure 36.1 in the cervical smear.

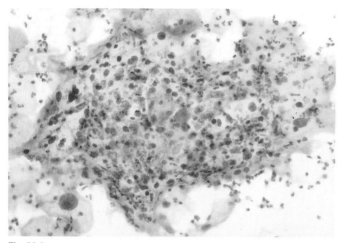

Fig. 36.1

◆ Question 36.1
What abnormalities do the nuclei of these cells show?

The report on the cervical smear from the pathology laboratory reads 'Severely dyskaryotic cells present, refer to a gynaecologist for further investigation and treatment'. The gynaecologist takes a biopsy from the cervix and as a result of the histopathological report on that specimen performs a hysterectomy. The hysterectomy specimen has the appearances shown in Figure 36.2.

◆ Answer 36.1
There is marked pleomorphism with some nuclear diameters more than twice that of other cells. The nuclei are also all much darker than would be expected (nuclear hyperchromatism).

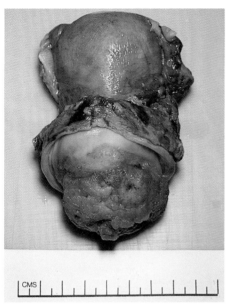

Fig. 36.2

◆ **Question 36.2**
What abnormality can be seen?

◆ **Question 36.3**
What is this lesion most likely to be?

The histopathologist takes samples from the lesion which has the microscopic appearances shown in Figure 36.3.

◆ **Answer 36.2**
There is an exophytic tumour of the cervix with an irregular surface.

◆ **Answer 36.3**
Squamous carcinoma of the cervix.

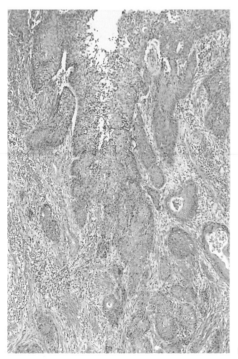

Fig. 36.3

◆ **Question 36.4**
Do these appearances confirm your diagnosis of the lesion?

Epithelium on the cervix adjacent to the squamous carcinoma had the appearances shown in Figure 36.4.

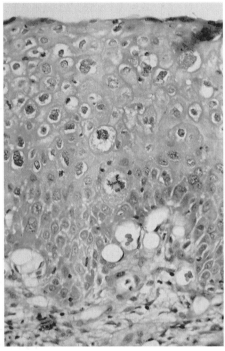

Fig. 36.4

◆ **Question 36.5**
What abnormalities are present in this epithelium?

◆ **Question 36.6**
Why might cervical smears taken at regular intervals have prevented the development of this squamous carcinoma?

◆ **Answer 36.4**
The picture shows a tumour which is invading the stromal tissue suggesting that it is a malignant neoplastic process. The tumour appears to be arising from the epithelial surface so it is a carcinoma (a malignant epithelial tumour). Examination at higher magnification would reveal evidence of squamous differentiation, keratin production and intercellular bridges.

◆ **Answer 36.5**
In a normal area of squamous epithelium there will be a well-organized architecture with a basal layer of cells which are mitotically active and then progressive change into keratinised cells at the surface. In this picture there are mitotic figures above the basal layer and some of these are abnormal (a tripolar mitotic figure is evident). The nuclei are not arranged regularly (loss of nuclear polarity) and are not maturing fully at the surface. These features combine to give the features of severe epithelial dysplasia which in the cervix will be classified as cervical intra-epithelial neoplasia grade 3 (CIN 3).

◆ **Answer 36.6**
Cervical cytology can detect dysplasia in the cervical epithelium which is manifest as dykaryotic cells on a cervical smear. Dysplasia is a premalignant condition in the cervix and marked degrees of dysplasia (CIN 3) often progress to invasive carcinomas but this usually takes place over a relatively long period of time. In the United Kingdom there is a national cervical screening programme which aims to detect dysplasia of the cervical epithelium which may then be treated by laser ablation, loop diathermy excision or (more rarely recently) cone biopsy.

◆ **Question 36.7**

Apart from the type of tumour what other information will the surgeon wish the histopathologist to include in the pathology report?

◆ **Question 36.8**

What are the risk factors for the development of cervical carcinoma and can you detect any of these in Figure 36.4?

Revision

■ Cytopathology, see pp. 68–70

■ Cervical cancer screening, see pp. 558–559

■ Carcinoma of the cervix, see pp. 556–560

■ Cervical intra-epithelial neoplasia, see p. 558

■ Human papillovirus, see pp. 215, 410, 448, 558–559, 602

◆ **Answer 36.7**

The stage of the tumour. The extent to which the tumour has spread is an important determinant of patient prognosis and may influence choice of treatment. The pathologist would sample the specimen to determine the size and depth of invasion of the cervical tumour, whether it is completely excised and whether any sampled lymph nodes contain metastatic carcinoma. Stage I cervical carcinoma is confined to the cervix, stage II extends beyond the cervix but not to the pelvic wall, stage III may extend onto the pelvic wall and/or the lower third of the vagina and stage IV indicates extension outside the reproductive tract. Once the tumour has metastasised to the para-aortic lymph nodes the prognosis is very poor.

◆ **Answer 36.8**

The risk factors include early age at first intercourse, frequency of intercourse and number of sexual partners. These factors would be consistent with an infectious agent transmitted by sexual intercourse and types of the human papillomaviruses (HPV) have been proposed as such agents. In Figure 36.4 there is histological evidence of HPV infection with cells with vacuolated cytoplasm (koilocytes). It is also clear that, as with the majority of human tumours, a single agent is not solely responsible for initiation/progression of the neoplastic process and other factors will be involved. Cigarette smoking is a risk factor which appears to be independent of HPV infection.

Loose stools

A 45-year-old married woman, a teacher in a school for children with learning difficulties, asks her doctor to visit her because she has had severe diarrhoea for the last week with episodes of abdominal pain. She has had diarrhoea occasionally before, but never as severe as this. This episode started 2 weeks after she had returned from staying with her daughter in Ireland; while in Ireland she developed a chest infection for which she received antibiotic treatment. On the day before the doctor's visit, she had six bouts of diarrhoea and she now feels weak and listless.

◆ **Question 37.1**
What are the main causes of diarrhoea?

The patient feels compelled to make another visit to the toilet during the doctor's visit. The doctor asks her not to flush the toilet, so the contents can be examined. The material in the toilet is stained with fresh blood.

The doctor contacts the local hospital and arranges for the patient's urgent admission. On admission, she has a thorough clinical examination. The patient is pale and obviously dehydrated. Her abdomen is slightly distended and tender.

◆ **Question 37.2**
What investigations should be performed?

◆ **Question 37.3**
What organisms should be looked for in a case of diarrhoea?

The microbiology report states that no bowel pathogenic organisms have been detected. The results of the other investigations are:

	Patient's values	Normal range
Sodium	148 mmol/l	130–147 mmol/l
Potassium	3.0 mmol/l	3.3–5.5 mmol/l
Urea	9.0 mmol/l	3.3–8.3 mmol/l
Creatinine	110 μmol/l	60–120 μmol/l
Haemoglobin	9.0 g/dl	11.5–15.5 g/dl

The total white cell count and differential are normal.

◆ **Question 37.4**
How do you interpret the results of these investigations?

◆ **Answer 37.1**
Diarrhoea is most commonly due to gastrointestinal infections ('food poisoning'), but most of these last for only a few days and remit spontaneously. Diarrhoea of the duration, frequency and severity in this patient may be due to primary non-infective disease of the gastrointestinal tract.

◆ **Answer 37.2**
Stool samples should be sent for microbiological investigations. The patient's electrolytes, haemoglobin and white cell count should also be checked.

◆ **Answer 37.3**
In children, many cases of diarrhoea are due to rotaviruses. In adults, depending on the country, diarrhoea may be due to bacteria such as toxigenic *Escherichia coli*, shigellae, or salmonellae, or to parasites such as pathogenic amoebae. Another possibility in this case is pseudomembranous colitis following antibiotic therapy; this is due to a toxin produced by *Clostridium difficile*.

◆ **Answer 37.4**
The cause of the diarrhoea is likely to be non-infective. The serum biochemistry is most consistent with dehydration (high sodium, urea and creatinine); the low serum potassium accounts for the patient's weakness and is due to potassium loss from the bowel. The anaemia is almost certainly due to blood loss.

The next investigation to be performed is colonoscopy. This reveals congested and ulcerated colonic and rectal mucosa. A biopsy is taken (Fig. 37.1).

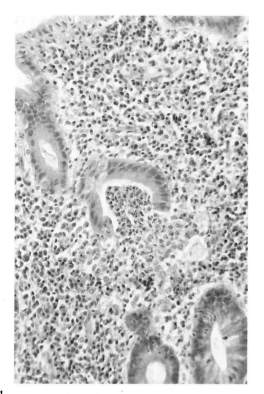

Fig. 37.1

◆ Question 37.5
What are the main abnormalities in the rectal biopsy and what is the most likely diagnosis?

The patient is treated with steroids and she improves rapidly. Within 3 weeks she is fit enough for further investigation. This includes radiological imaging of the small and large intestine: the small intestine is normal, but the colon shows a loss of haustral pattern throughout the transverse and descending colon.

◆ Question 37.6
Is Crohn's disease or ulcerative colitis more likely?

The patient is told that she has ulcerative colitis. The current exacerbation responds to treatment, but the patient is told that the problem may recur.

During the next 5 years the patient has several further exacerbations of the condition; she develops profuse diarrhoea with blood loss resulting in iron deficiency anaemia. Her treatment is changed, but the attacks continue intermittently.

◆ Answer 37.5
The biopsy shows a dense inflammatory infiltrate in the lamina propria and infiltration of the gland crypts by neutrophil polymorphs (crypt abscesses). The glands are also distorted. These appearances are most likely to be due to chronic inflammatory bowel disease (ulcerative colitis or Crohn's disease).

◆ Answer 37.6
Ulcerative colitis. There is nothing to favour Crohn's disease in this case: the abnormalities seem confined to the colon and no granulomas were seen in the biopsy.

After 10 years, during a quiescent period of the disease, she has a colonoscopic biopsy, the report on which refers to the presence of low-grade dysplasia.

◆ Question 37.7
What is the significance of low-grade dysplasia in this patient?

At this time the patient also has blood taken for haematological and biochemical investigations. She is found to be slightly anaemic, but the liver biochemistry tests reveal:

	Patient's values	Normal range
Bilirubin	25 μmol/l	5–147 μmol/l
Aspartate aminotransferase (AST)	50 U/l	5–40 U/l
Alanine aminotransferase (ALT)	45 U/l	5–40 U/l
Gamma glutamyltransferase	60 U/l	0–65 U/l
Alkaline phosphatase	620 U/l	30–110 U/l

◆ Question 37.8
What is the significance of these biochemical abnormalities?

The patient's ulcerative colitis becomes unresponsive to medical treatment. She is persistently anaemic and losing weight. In view of this, and the biopsy evidence of dysplasia and suspicion of sclerosing cholangitis, she is advised to have a total colectomy. This is done and the colon shows extensive ulceration, but no evidence of carcinoma.
The patient makes a good post-operative recovery.

Revision

- Electrolyte homeostasis, see pp. 149–150
- Ulcerative colitis, see pp. 435–437
- Preneoplastic lesions, see p. 273
- Dysplasia, see pp. 108, 254

◆ Answer 37.7
Patients with chronic ulcerative colitis have an increased risk of developing carcinoma of the colon. For this reason, such patients often have routine colonoscopic biopsies to look for dysplasia; patients with dysplasia in their colonoscopic biopsies have the greatest risk of developing colonic carcinoma. Low-grade dysplasia is not sufficient to justify surgical intervention, but the condition should be monitored by regular colonoscopy and biopsy.

◆ Answer 37.8
The combination of a high alkaline phosphatase and an elevated bilirubin is indicative of a biliary obstructive lesion, even if the patient does not appear to be jaundiced. In the context of chronic ulcerative colitis, the most likely cause is sclerosing cholangitis; there is an increased incidence of this rare condition in patients with ulcerative colitis. In this condition the small intrahepatic bile ducts become obstructed and eventually destroyed by fibrous tissue proliferation.

Increasing girth

A 44-year-old woman attends her general practitioner's surgery where she tells the doctor that she has noticed that her abdomen appears distended and her weight has increased by 3 kg. The GP does not think that the patient looks overweight at all but the patient explains that she is an enthusiastic distance runner who keeps a careful watch on her weight. She also says that when out running she sometimes feels a dragging sensation in her lower abdomen. On examination the GP finds that the patient's general physical condition is good and the only abnormality, on bimanual abdominovaginal examination, is a fullness in the left iliac fossa. The GP refers her to a gynaecologist at the local hospital. At the hospital an ultrasound scan reveals a mass which is contiguous with the left ovary. This lesion is removed by the gynaecologist at a laparotomy and has the external appearances shown in Figure 38.1. The fallopian tube is visible stretched across the top of the lesion.

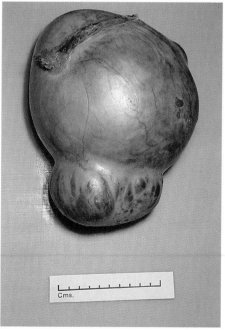

Fig. 38.1

◆ **Question 38.1**
Do these external macroscopic appearances give any clues as to whether this lesion is benign or malignant?

◆ **Answer 38.1**
The external surface is smooth with no obvious external tumour tissue which favours a benign tumour.

When the lesion is sliced in the pathology laboratory it has the appearances shown in Figure 38.2.

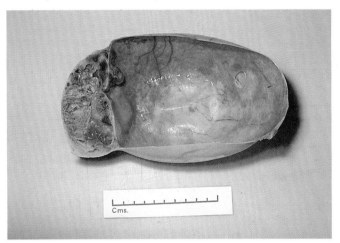

Fig. 38.2

◆ Question 38.2
Does the internal appearance give any clues as to whether this lesion is benign or malignant?

A representative area of the wall of the cyst shows the microscopic appearance shown in Figure 38.3 (the histopathologist took many samples from the wall at a rate of one sample per 10 mm diameter of the cyst).

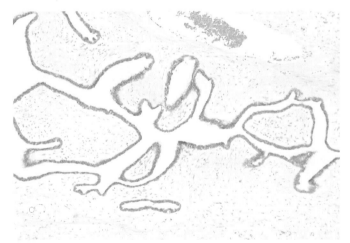

Fig. 38.3

◆ Question 38.3
Do these microscopic appearances confirm the benign nature of the neoplastic process?

◆ Question 38.4
What benign tumours of the ovary are there?

◆ Answer 38.2
The cut surface shows that the lesion is cystic rather than solid and is a single cyst (unilocular) rather than multiple cysts. No areas of solid papillary tissue are evident macroscopically, the solid tissue on the left of the picture is the residual ovary. These appearances are again in favour of a benign lesion but histological examination by a histopathologist must be performed before a definitive assessment can be made.

◆ Answer 38.3
Yes. The picture shows pink-staining stromal tissue with a blue-staining lining of epithelial cells. The epithelial cells are in a single layer and there is no evidence of invasion of the stromal tissue. Examination of the tissue at higher magnification showed that the epithelial cells had nuclei that were all a similar size (there was no significant nuclear pleomorphism) and were not unduly dark (no significant hyperchromatism). All these features combine to confirm the benign nature of the lesion.

◆ Answer 38.4
When considering the possible tumours that can arise in an organ it is helpful to consider the types of tissue that are present. In the ovary there is epithelial tissue (which is mainly glandular), stromal tissue and germ cells. The benign tumours that may occur thus include adenomas, fibromas/thecomas, and mature cystic teratomas (derived from germ cells).

◆ Question 38.5

Can you give a more precise name for this tumour?

✕ Malignant tumours of the ovary will include those derived from the epithelium (carcinomas), germ cells (immature teratoma, dysgerminoma, choriocarcinoma and yolk sac tumour) and metastatic tumours (such as gastric carcinoma producing Krukenberg tumours). Ovarian carcinoma in England and Wales caused death in 83% of women in whom it was diagnosed, whereas carcinoma of the cervix caused death in 54% of women in whom it was diagnosed.

◆ Question 38.6

What anatomical and pathological explanations can you give for these differences in mortality?

Revision

- ■ Tumour shape and behaviour, see pp. 248–250
- ■ Ovarian tumours, see pp. 570–576

◆ Answer 38.5

This tumour is composed of benign epithelial cells, the cyst was filled with a serous fluid and at high magnification the cells appear ciliated without mucin vacuoles. The precise type of this tumour is thus a benign serous cystadenoma.

◆ Answer 38.6

Anatomically the ovaries lie in the peritoneal cavity and are not easily examined, they can increase in size without detection especially in obese subjects. The cervix projects into the vagina which may be examined quite easily. In the cervix there is a well-characterised sequence of preneoplastic dysplasia arising and progressing to invasive carcinoma over a long period of time, screening by cervical cytology is designed to interrupt the sequence before the onset of invasion. A preneoplastic sequence in the ovary has not been identified and no screening programme is available.

'Her throat is better but now she's got a rash'

A 11-year-old girl is brought back to your surgery by her mother. Three weeks ago you saw the girl when she had a sore throat. You prescribed a course of antibiotics (ampicillin) in view of pyrexia and tonsillar enlargement. On further questioning, you discover that she has abdominal pain, is listless and unwell, and has pain in her joints. Her throat is better but now she's got a rash.

◆ **Question 39.1**
What are the leading diagnoses at this stage?

You check the patient's notes and find that the throat swab that you took at presentation 3 weeks ago yielded no growth in the microbiology laboratory.

◆ **Question 39.2**
What are the points in your symptomatic enquiry to which you should pay particular attention?

Your enquiries reveal that the antibiotics have been taken correctly, that the joint and abdominal pains came on at approximately the same time and that her mother has switched to a new brand of washing powder in a compact box and that she wonders whether this has caused the rash. The girl is concerned that excess hockey practice may have led to the joint pains.

◆ **Question 39.3**
What are the main points to note on examination?

◆ **Question 39.4**
On examining the skin (Fig. 39.1) and mucous membranes (Fig. 39.2), how would you classify the rash?

◆ **Answer 39.1**
Rheumatic fever (due to the history of previous upper respiratory tract infection which may have been streptococcal, and which produces a rash and arthralgia), drug related rashes (including erythema multiforme, possibly following the course of antibiotics, and the interaction of glandular fever with ampicillin which is notorious for producing rashes), and Henoch-Schönlein purpura (a rare type of anaphylactoid purpura which can follow infections in children).

◆ **Answer 39.2**
You need to find out whether the antibiotics were in fact taken, more about the timing and distribution of the joint pains, whether there has been any chest pain, follow up the mention of abdominal pain with enquiry about the stools, particularly whether blood has been present, ask about the urine to ascertain how the amount compares with normal and whether there has been any change in its appearance.

◆ **Answer 39.3**
The girl has potentially serious disease so thorough examination is needed. However, examination should first focus on the rash, the cardiovascular system, the abdomen and the joints.

◆ **Answer 39.4**
The rash is purpuric, that is to say, characterised by areas of haemorrhage into the skin.

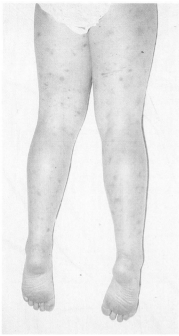

Fig. 39.1

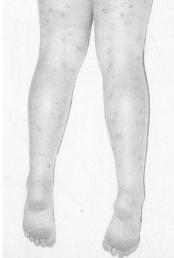

Fig. 39.2

On examination you find an ill-looking child who is apyrexial and apart from the rash the only abnormal physical signs are mild hypertension at 140/85 mmHg, a slightly tender abdomen and tender knee joints.

◆ **Question 39.5**
What is the most important test to do next in your surgery?

The practice nurse and patient return with a flask of slightly frothy mildly cloudy urine. You do not have facilities for urine microscopy so you perform one of the commercially-available combined stick tests. This shows no evidence of glycosuria but heavy albuminuria and a trace of haematuria.

◆ **Question 39.6**
What should you do next?

The hospital doctors repeat your history taking and examination and arrange urgent blood tests, radiographs of the chest, abdomen and affected joints, and send off urine for microscopy, culture and protein estimation. The blood count and film are normal, but there is moderate elevation of the blood urea and creatinine and a little depression of the albumin. The urine contains hyaline and granular casts and its protein content is 3g/l.

◆ **Answer 39.5**
You should examine and test a freshly passed urine sample.

◆ **Answer 39.6**
The patient has evidence of renal damage (hypertension, albuminuria, haematuria). You telephone the paediatric firm on call: the senior house officer shares your concerns and arranges immediate admission.

◆ Question 39.7
What do these findings tell you?

The consultant nephrologist visits and decides to perform a renal biopsy under ultrasound guidance.

◆ Question 39.8
What additional blood tests should be done first?

You attend the renal biopsy conference two days later where the histopathologist demonstrates the biopsy to you. The haematoxylin and eosin stained renal biopsy is shown in Figure 39.3 and direct immunofluorescence of this for IgA is shown in Figure 39.4.

◆ Answer 39.7
The patient is in acute renal failure with proteinuria falling just short of nephrotic syndrome.

◆ Answer 39.8
Renal biopsy is an invasive procedure with a risk of haemorrhage. The patient's platelet count is already known from the full blood count, but blood should be sent for grouping and saving and screening tests of the coagulation factors must be performed.

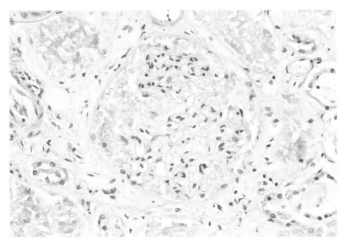

Fig. 39.3

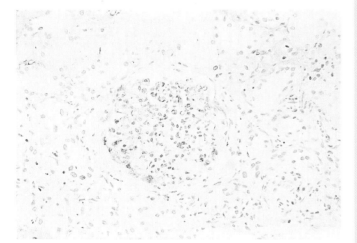

Fig. 39.4

◆ Question 39.9

What is the structure shown in Figure 39.3? What is the point of the immunofluorescence study?

All of the glomeruli in this case show widespread mesangial deposits of IgA. The histopathologist points out that this is a very distinctive finding and coupled with the history of previous sore throat, purpuric skin rash, joint and abdominal pains is diagnostic of Henoch-Schönlein purpura. Establishing a specific diagnosis in this way was extremely useful. Although there is no specific treatment, you know that most patients with this uncommon condition have a good prognosis. The patient, after requiring temporary haemodialysis for a period of 2 weeks, makes a full recovery and is discharged home after 3 weeks without any evidence of renal impairment.

Revision

- Rheumatic fever, see pp. 814–815
- Determining bacterial sensitivity to antibiotics, see pp. 73–74
- Glomerular disease, see pp. 626–740
- Post-streptococcal glomerulonephritis, see pp. 631–632
- Nephrotic syndrome, see p. 628

◆ Answer 39.9

This is a glomerulus. Not being familiar with looking at these regularly, you cannot see anything wrong with it. The histopathologist points out that it shows areas of hypercellularity within all of the glomeruli typical of focal proliferative glomerulonephritis. Immunofluorescence enables deposits of immunoglobulins, fibrin and complement components to be identified specifically within the glomerulus.

A lump in the armpit

A 43-year-old woman presents to her general practitioner with a lump in her left armpit. The lump has appeared over a period of 3 months and is getting larger. She was scratched by her neighbour's cat a few weeks before the lump became evident. Her health is otherwise good. The general practitioner examines her and finds a firm but mobile lump in the left axilla which is 20 mm in diameter. There is an old healed scar on the left side of the chest. This lesion (Fig. 40.1) was removed from the breast 2 years previously and at the edge of this lesion the microscopic appearances in Figure 40.2 were present.

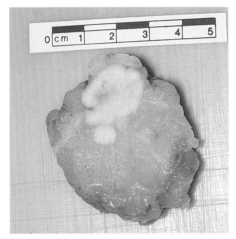

Fig. 40.1

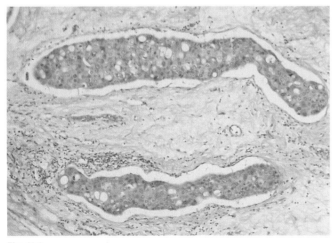

Fig. 40.2

◆ **Question 40.1**
What differential diagnosis can you give for the lump in the left axilla?

◆ **Answer 40.1**
Infective causes especially cat scratch fever (given the history), metastatic breast carcinoma, lymphoma.

◆ Question 40.2
What procedures could give a definitive diagnosis?

The patient is referred to the local hospital and the lump is excised by a surgeon. The histopathological report says: 'This lymph node is largely replaced by metastatic adenocarcinoma of similar appearance to the previously excised breast carcinoma.'

◆ Question 40.3
Which other groups of lymph nodes can breast carcinoma metastasise to?

◆ Question 40.4
What percentage of women with breast carcinoma have axillary lymph node metastases at the time of presentation?

◆ Question 40.5
In which part of the lymph node do metastases first appear?

◆ Question 40.6
Lymph node metastasis is an adverse prognostic factor in breast carcinoma. What other known adverse prognostic factors are there?

Revision

■ Lymphadenopathy, see pp. 659–674

■ Metastasis, see pp. 284–287

■ Breast cancer prognosis, see pp. 547–549

◆ Answer 40.2
Cytological examination of a fine-needle aspirate of the lump could give a diagnosis but the architecture of a lymph node cannot be assessed in such material and it is difficult to diagnose some pathologies. Excision of the lump and submission for histological examination should produce a definitive diagnosis.

◆ Answer 40.3
Intramammary, supraclavicular and those associated with internal mammary vessels.

◆ Answer 40.4
Between 40 and 50%.

◆ Answer 40.5
The marginal sinus.

◆ Answer 40.6
Poor differentiation, negative oestrogen receptor status, blood-borne metastases.

An iatrogenic black toe

A 56-year-old insurance broker is referred to a cardiologist by his general practitioner. The patient gives a long history of chest pain associated with exercise. Initially the pain came on during the 17th and 18th holes of a round of golf but more recently it appeared as early as the 5th hole. The purchase of a motorised golf bag trolley has enabled him to reach the 9th hole but he cannot complete a whole round because of the severity of the chest pain. His past medical history shows he had a hernia repair 5 years previously and knee ligament repair when he was 32 years, following an injury sustained on the rugby field. He says that he finds his job is stressful with worries about large claims in some areas of the insurance market but he is financially secure at present. He used to smoke 20 cigarettes a day but 5 years ago gave up cigarette smoking and changed to cigars. On examination the cardiologist finds a moderately obese man with no abnormalities apart from a quiet carotid bruit on the left side; pedal pulses are easily detected on both sides.

◆ **Question 41.1**
What is the most probable cause of his chest pain?

◆ **Question 41.2**
What risk factors does the patient have for atherosclerosis?

The cardiologist sends the patient for an exercise electrocardiographic test which shows elevation of ST segments on exercise and confirms the diagnosis of ischaemic heart disease. The patient then has coronary artery angiography performed to assess whether surgery or angioplasty could be used to improve blood flow within the coronary arteries. Angiography shows a tight stenosis in the proximal part of the left anterior descending artery which could be bypassed by grafting. 36 hours after the angiography the patient complains of pain in his left foot; on examination two of his toes show gangrenous change but the pedal pulses are present. The condition of the toes does not improve and they are amputated. Histological examination of the toes reveals the appearances shown in Figure 41.1.

◆ **Answer 41.1**
Angina pectoris due to coronary artery atherosclerosis.

◆ **Answer 41.2**
Cigarette smoking is the most important factor in this patient. Moderate obesity and a stressful occupation might be considered to be minor risk factors for atherosclerosis. We have not been given information about his cholesterol and lipid levels or any family history of ischaemic heart disease.

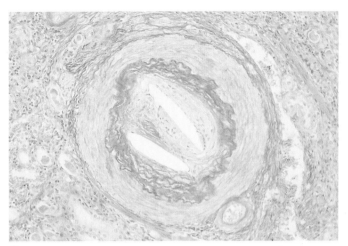

Fig. 41.1

◆ **Question 41.3**
What abnormal changes can you see in the blood vessels?

◆ **Question 41.4**
What is this material and how has it reached the vessels in the toes?

◆ **Question 41.5**
What other organs could these crystals have embolised to and what complications could result?

Revision

■ Ischaemic heart disease, see pp. 335–339

■ Embolism, see pp. 169–173

chol. clefts !

◆ **Answer 41.3**
The lumen of the blood vessel contains needle-shaped clefts which would have contained material which has dissolved during histological processing. Around these clefts there is a giant cell reaction. There is no evidence of an arteritis.

◆ **Answer 41.4**
The needle-shaped clefts contained cholesterol crystals which had embolised from atheromatous plaques in the aorta when these were disrupted by the tip of the catheter during angiography.

◆ **Answer 41.5**
The cholesterol crystals could have embolised to any organs distal to the disrupted atheromatous plaque. Since the large ulcerated atheromatous plaques are often in the abdominal aorta these organs include the kidneys, spleen and intestine. In the kidneys multiple cholesterol emboli can cause renal failure by ischaemic damage. In the intestine ischaemia due to cholesterol embolism may produce fibrous strictures.

Pyrexia of unknown origin

A 44-year-old man presents with a 1-month history of waking up at night drenched in sweat, loss of about 4 kg weight and back ache. He has recently returned from holiday in the Bahamas, where he took no anti-malarial prophylactics.

On examination, he is pale, looks ill, has a temperature of 39°C and is tender over the lumbar spine.

◆ Question 42.1
What initial investigations should be done?

No malarial parasites are seen. The urine shows microscopic haematuria, the liver function tests show elevation of the transaminases, the blood count shows elevation of the haematocrit and the erythrocyte sedimentation rate (ESR) is 84 mm per hour. The patient is still pyrexial.

◆ Question 42.2
What do all these abnormal findings mean?

You refer the patient to hospital where ultrasound examination of the renal/urinary system is performed. A mass is seen at the upper pole of the left kidney.

◆ Question 42.3
In the context of the patient's abnormal findings, what is the most likely nature of the mass?

The patient's lumbar spine radiograph shows a lucent lesion in L3 (Fig. 42.1).

◆ Answer 42.1
This is an investigation of pyrexia of unknown origin. The patient needs a thick blood film to look for malarial parasites, blood and urine cultures, brucella titres, full blood count, liver function tests and a chest radiograph.

◆ Answer 42.2
Most are very non-specific. The elevated ESR confirms that the patient is ill and points to an inflammatory, infective or neoplastic process. The abnormal liver function tests indicate liver parenchymal damage which could be due to a multitude of causes. Only the haematuria points to a specific system.

◆ Answer 42.3
A renal cell carcinoma would explain malaise, abnormal liver function tests, pyrexia of unknown origin, haematuria and elevation of the haematocrit.

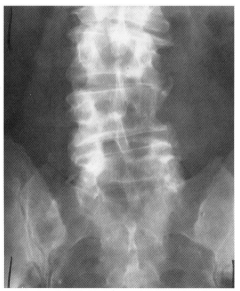

Fig. 42.1

◆ **Question 42.4**
What is this likely to be?

◆ **Question 42.5**
If the patient has a metastasis, is there any point in excising the primary tumour?

The patient undergoes left radical nephrectomy through a midline abdominal incision.

◆ **Question 42.6**
Why is the kidney not removed through a loin incision?

Figure 42.2 shows the nephrectomy specimen.

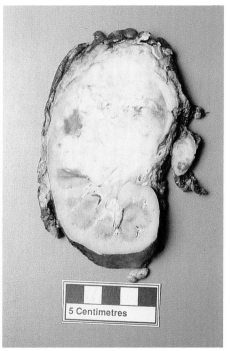

Fig. 42.2

◆ **Answer 42.4**
It is likely to be a metastasis of renal cell carcinoma.

◆ **Answer 42.5**
Usually the answer to this is 'no'. In the case of renal cell carcinoma, however, patients sometimes have prolonged survival after excision of the primary tumour and radiotherapy to an apparently solitary metastasis. The tumour is notoriously unpredictable in behaviour.

◆ **Answer 42.6**
The renal vein needs to be clamped before the kidney is mobilised to prevent tumour seeding via the venous drainage.

◆ **Question 42.7**
What are the prognostic features to look for in the specimen?

◆ **Answer 42.7**
Large size of the tumour, capsular penetration, macroscopic venous invasion and involvement of lymph nodes (if there are any) at the renal hilum are adverse prognostic features.

Figure 42.3 shows a section taken from the vascular pedicle of the kidney.

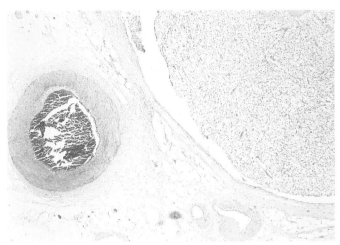

Fig. 42.3

◆ **Question 42.8**
What does this show?

Patients with venous invasion by renal cell carcinoma have a very poor prognosis, with only 15–20% 5-year survival. The tumour is notorious for its ability to invade veins and spread through the blood stream. Sometimes a large cord of tumour grows into the inferior vena cava and reaches the right atrium or embolises to the lungs.

Revision

■ Renal cell carcinoma, see pp. 650–651

■ Invasion, see pp. 283–284

■ Metastasis, see pp. 284–287

◆ **Answer 42.8**
It shows a large vein consistent with the renal vein plugged by clear cell adenocarcinoma, typical of renal cell carcinoma.

Nipple discharge

A 45-year-old woman presents to your outpatient clinic with a 1-month history of nipple discharge. On questioning, she says that it is red-brown coloured and present every day. She has had three pregnancies, the last when she was 37, and breast-fed the babies.

◆ **Question 43.1**
Are there any special points to note in questioning her?

Further questioning reveals that she received a prescription for depression 2 years ago, but that she is now well and taking no medication.

◆ **Question 43.2**
What is the differential diagnosis for the nipple discharge?

On examination, both breasts are generally lumpy. There is no lymph node enlargement. The visual fields are normal.

◆ **Question 43.3**
What is the point of assessing the visual fields?

You express some bloody discharge from the nipple and send it for cytology.

◆ **Question 43.4**
Is this a useful investigation?

◆ **Answer 43.1**
You need to consider whether she might be pregnant, consider endocrine disease and take an accurate history of drug consumption.

◆ **Answer 43.2**
This includes intraduct papilloma, duct ectasia, fibrocystic disease, breast carcinoma, hormonal effects such as pregnancy, pituitary tumours and drug effects such as phenothiazines which act via the hypothalamus on the pituitary causing it to secrete prolactin.

◆ **Answer 43.3**
To exclude visual field defects due to pituitary tumours.

◆ **Answer 43.4**
No. Nipple discharge tends to contain blood and degenerate cells only; very rarely can any diagnosis be made on it.

Mammography (Fig. 43.1) shows bilateral fibrocystic disease only. The surgeon recommends to the patient that the breast duct and lactiferous sinus responsible be excised for histology and that further treatment may be needed depending on the result. The lesion is most likely to be benign but histology is the only way to exclude malignancy.

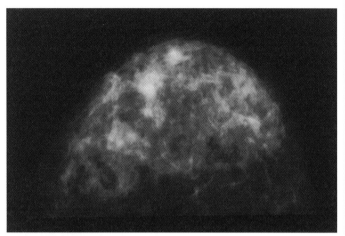

Fig. 43.1

◆ **Question 43.5**
Because of the uncertainty of the diagnosis, couldn't the surgeon ask for intra-operative frozen section diagnosis?

The patient's breast looks like Figure 43.2 after surgery.

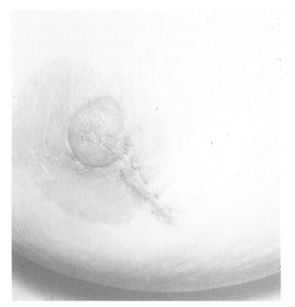

Fig. 43.2

◆ **Answer 43.5**
No. Lesions that cause nipple discharge are likely to be intraduct papillary growths which require extensive sampling and careful assessment on paraffin sections. They are not suitable for frozen section diagnosis.

◆ **Question 43.6**
What has she had done?

Figure 43.3 shows the histology of the excised breast duct.

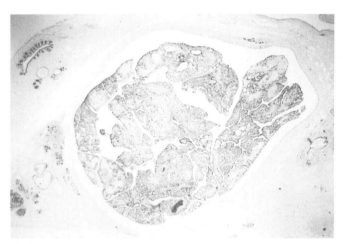

Fig. 43.3

◆ **Question 43.7**
What abnormality can you see?

The patient's histopathology report reads: 'This contains a benign intraduct papilloma without evidence of malignancy. Excision appears complete.'
The patient makes a complete recovery and is discharged from follow-up.

Revision

■ Pituitary neoplasms, see pp. 490–491

■ Cytopathology, see pp. 68–70

■ Breast duct papilloma, see p. 532

◆ **Answer 43.6**
Radial and circumferential scars around the nipple like this are seen after microdochectomy, which involves cannulation of the discharging breast duct from the nipple and local excision.

◆ **Answer 43.7**
There is a growth of ductal epithelium and fibrovascular tissue into the distended duct.

'He just grabbed the teapot by the spout'

A 3-year-old child is brought into Accident and Emergency by his mother with a history of scalding. The accident happened in the hospital canteen at the end of visiting time and the mother ran directly to the department.

◆ Question 44.1
What is appropriate first aid?

On examination the child has an area of erythema with small blisters on the right cheek, right shoulder and right arm and hand. There is a 2-cm white area within the chest erythema.

◆ Question 44.2
What factors will determine whether or not there will be permanent damage?

◆ Question 44.3
What physiological processes will have already begun in the wound?

The child is treated, the wounds dressed and the child referred to a burns unit. At 5 days the face is still reddened but seems to be healing. The white area on the chest has now turned black and sloughs off revealing a red friable tissue that bleeds easily.

◆ Question 44.4
What is this tissue and what is the main risk at this stage?

◆ Answer 44.1
In the first 10 to 15 minutes of a burn the dermal temperature remains quite high and it is worth trying to limit damage by lowering this with ice packs to the affected area. Domestically packets of frozen peas are very good because they can be moulded to the area of the burn.

◆ Answer 44.2
The depth of the burn will determine the eventual outcome. In superficial burns the damage is limited to the epidermis and papillary dermis. Since the blood vessels are not destroyed and the blood in the area is not coagulated, blistering can occur and this is generally a good sign. Even if the epidermis is killed the epidermal adnexae which project downwards are spared and these can provide cells to repopulate the surface. The deeper the burn the less chance there is of this happening. Scarring develops when the deeper dermis is damaged and when re-epithelialization is delayed.

◆ Answer 44.3
The reddened area is a sign of inflammation. The early phase of this process is vascular dilatation which accounts for the redness. Consequently a white area within a burn may mean that the vessels are destroyed and that this area is more badly damaged and cannot respond with the adaptive and essential process of inflammation. In these areas new skin cannot be regenerated and the repair process of fibrosis and scarring will occur. The most difficult problem with this is that the scar tissue will contract markedly and can cause severe deformity.

◆ Answer 44.4
This is granulation tissue. The little friable 'granules' are loops of capillaries and are nothing to do with granulomas.

In the burns unit there is a patient with 80% of his skin surface burnt in an accident that occurred whilst he was welding a petrol tank. He walked into the Accident and Emergency department the day before and seems to be feeling no pain.

◆ Question 44.5
What is his prognosis?

◆ Question 44.6
What non-clinical action should you also take after dealing with the immediate clinical problem of the child?

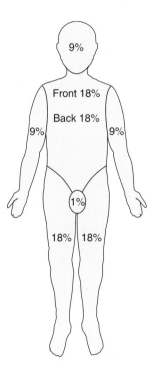

9%

Front 18%

Back 18%

9% 9%

1%

18% | 18%

Fig. 44.1

Revision

- Skin healing, see pp. 91–92, 121–123
- Granulation tissue, see p. 121
- Skin as a barrier, see pp. 749–750
- Acute inflammation, see pp. 222–236

On the basis of this granulation tissue epithelial cells from the viable edges of the wound and from remaining adnexal structures such as hair follicles and sweat glands, will grow out and eventually re-epithelialize the wound. Since the epithelium has been lost then one of its functions, the prevention of infection, has also been lost. If infection occurs it delays healing, produces a greater degree of scarring and may cause severe systemic problems. Prevention of infection is of primary concern in the treatment of any trauma in which the integrity of the skin is lost.

◆ Answer 44.5
The lack of pain and lesser sensation in burns is an ominous sign since it indicates that the burn is deep enough to have destroyed the dermal nerves. This means that the full thickness of skin is dead and will eventually slough leaving a large area of body surface unprotected against fluid and electrolyte loss and the ingress of micro-organisms. Ten to 15% skin loss will require immediate transfusion and active treatment for shock as well as antibiotic cover. Eighty % skin loss will be fatal in most cases, but smaller areas of skin loss in the very young and in those over 40 years of age can also be fatal. Figure 44.1 shows the method of calculating percentages (rule of nine). Remember that the proportions are different in children.

◆ Answer 44.6
Since the accident to the child occurred within the hospital it may be that the Trust has some legal liability and it would be sensible to inform chief executive's office as soon as possible. Obviously under such delicate circumstances it would be inappropriate for you to start advising the patient of their legal rights, or to suggest that they think of bringing an action against the hospital, or even apologizing for the accident which might have been entirely the fault of the mother. Such things are best dealt with formally by management.

CASE 45

. . . And do no harm

A 58-year-old solicitor goes to see his general practitioner complaining of shortness of breath. The patient says that he has always been a keen sportsman and has continued to play tennis twice a week for the past 2 years. He finds that playing doubles is tolerable but when playing singles he becomes very breathless and has to take long pauses for breath at the end of sustained rallies. On questioning he says that the breathlessness is most noticeable after about 10 minutes of exercise and then seems to ease. As a child he suffered from eczema but has had no other significant illnesses and has never smoked cigarettes. The GP measures the man's peak expiratory flow rate (PEFR) and finds it to be below normal.

◆ **Question 45.1**
What may his breathlessness be due to?

The GP prescribes a salbutamol inhaler and asks the patient to return in 2 months. On his return the patient says that initially the medication seemed to produce an improvement in the symptoms but that recently the breathlessness has got worse and he can only play doubles tennis. The GP refers the patient to a chest physician at the local hospital. On examination the chest physician finds a man who is slightly breathless at rest but otherwise appears healthy. On auscultation of the chest there are a few crackles but no wheezes are heard. A chest radiograph shows patchy shadowing in both lung fields. The chest physician arranges for the patient to attend the day case unit for a fibreoptic bronchoscopy. A transbronchial biopsy is taken at the bronchoscopy and the histopathological report of the specimen is:

> Macroscopic appearances:
> Two pieces of tissue each 2 mm in diameter.
>
> Microscopic appearances:
> Sections show alveolar lung tissue which shows proliferation of type II pneumocytes and some fibrosis. Alveolar macrophages are present in increased numbers. There is no evidence of malignancy and no alcohol-acid-fast bacilli are identified. The appearances are those of non-specific inflammation with fibrosis.

With the knowledge of this report, together with the clinical findings and the chest radiographs, the chest physician makes a working diagnosis of desquamative interstitial pneumonitis.

◆ **Question 45.2**
Which disease group does desquamative interstitial pneumonitis belong to?

◆ **Answer 45.1**
Breathlessness may be due to both pulmonary and cardiac causes. In this case the breathlessness has symptoms that could be compatible with exercise-induced asthma.

◆ **Answer 45.2**
Desquamative interstitial pneumonitis is one of the diseases within the fibrosing alveolitis group which itself is one of the groups within chronic interstitial lung diseases.

The chest physician prescribes corticosteroids which have been shown to produce benefit in halting or reducing the speed of progression of desquamative interstitial pneumonitis. Initially the patient shows some response and becomes less breathless but over the next 12 months the patient becomes more breathless and finally dies during a hospital admission for respiratory failure. Consent for an autopsy is obtained from the patient's relatives.

Figure 42.1 shows the macroscopic appearance of the lungs at autopsy, and Figure 45.2 the microscopic appearance of the lungs at autopsy.

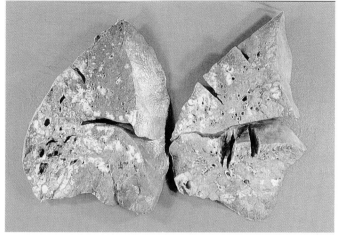

Fig. 45.1

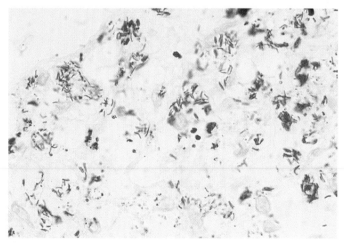

Fig. 45.2

◆ **Question 45.3**
What is the diagnosis?

◆ **Question 45.4**
What is the stain in Figure 45.2?

◆ **Answer 45.3**
Tuberculosis. Alcohol-acid-fast bacilli are present in Figure 45.2.

◆ **Answer 45.4**
Ziehl-Neelsen.

◆ **Question 45.5**

What investigation should be carried out to confirm the diagnosis?

◆ **Question 45.6**

What effect will the treatment for the working diagnosis of desquamative interstitial pneumonitis have had on the progression of the disease?

◆ **Question 45.7**

Can you offer an explanation for the temporary improvement in the patient's condition with the administration of steroids?

Revision

■ Interstitial lung disease, see pp. 389–393

■ Tuberculosis, see pp. 376–378

◆ **Answer 45.5**

Culture of the organism from the lung tissue.

◆ **Answer 45.6**

The steroids will have produced immunosupression which will have reduced the host resistance to the tuberculosis and speeded the progression of the disease.

◆ **Answer 45.7**

Much of the damage caused by tuberculosis is due to the immune response against the organism. This response will be reduced by the steroids producing an apparent improvement but at the expense of greater proliferation by the organism.

Opportunities for infection

A 28-year-old female presents to her general practitioner with complaints of tiredness, lethargy and a spotty rash around her ankles. The GP takes a blood sample and the results return:

	Patient's result	Normal range
Haemoglobin	6 g/dl	11.5–15.5 g/dl
White cell count	15×10^9/l	$4–11 \times 10^9$/l
Neutrophil count	0.5×10^9/l	$2.5–7.5 \times 10^9$/l
Platelets	30×10^9/l	$150–400 \times 10^9$/l

◆ **Question 46.1**
What sort of process could produce these results?

◆ **Question 46.2**
What is the red spotty rash on the patient's ankles likely to be due to?

The GP sends the patient immediately to the haematologists at the local hospital. The haematologists perform a bone marrow biopsy which shows that the patient has acute myeloblastic leukaemia. The patient is given transfusions of blood and platelets and is started on chemotherapy. After a week of treatment the blood results are:

	Patient's result	Normal range
Haemoglobin	11 g/dl	11.5–15.5 g/dl
White cell count	1.5×10^9/l	$4–11 \times 10^9$/l
Neutrophil count	$<0.1 \times 10^9$/l	$2.5–7.5 \times 10^9$/l
Platelets	40×10^9/l	$150–400 \times 10^9$/l

◆ **Question 46.3**
Is the leukaemia responding to the chemotherapy?

After 8 days of treatment the patient becomes breathless.

◆ **Question 46.4**
What is the most probable pathological cause for this breathlessness?

◆ **Answer 46.1**
There is anaemia and thrombocytopenia so there could be a global failure of the bone marrow to produce cells as is seen in aplastic anaemia but in this case the white cell count is raised. Although the nature of the white cells is not described in the results the neutrophil count is low so the most likely possibility is that there is a neoplastic proliferation of white cells which is replacing other elements within the bone marrow.

◆ **Answer 46.2**
Purpura due to the thrombocytopenia.

◆ **Answer 46.3**
Yes. The haemoglobin and platelet values will be changed by the transfusions but the white cell count has fallen which suggests that the leukaemia cells are being destroyed by the chemotherapy. A more accurate assessment of the response would be made by bone marrow biopsies at regular intervals during treatment.

◆ **Answer 46.4**
Breathlessness may be due to many causes mainly centred on cardiac or pulmonary pathology. At this time in the treatment the results for the patient's haemoglobin are at the lower end of the normal range so the breathlessness is unlikely to be due to anaemia. The patient is young and was fit prior to the development of the leukaemia so a coexistent cardiac pathology is unlikely and since it is early in the treatment period cardiac toxicity from the chemotherapy is improbable. The patient's neutrophil count is low so a cause which must be considered probable, and is important because it is treatable, is pulmonary infection.

◆ Question 46.5
What investigations should be performed?

Specimens for culture and sensitivities are obtained and the patient is started on broad-spectrum antibiotic therapy pending the results of these tests. Culture does not grow any bacterial organisms and the patient's breathlessness has become worse.

◆ Question 46.6
What other infective causes should be considered?

Antifungal agents are added to the patient's therapy but her condition deteriorates and she dies. The haematologists complete the death certificate giving acute myeloblastic leukaemia as the cause of death and they obtain permission for an autopsy from the deceased's relatives.

◆ Question 46.7
Since the clinicians know the cause of death why do they request an autopsy examination?

Figure 46.1 shows the lesions seen on the pleural surfaces at autopsy. Figure 46.2 shows the macroscopic appearance of the lungs and Figure 46.3 shows what microscopic examination reveals.

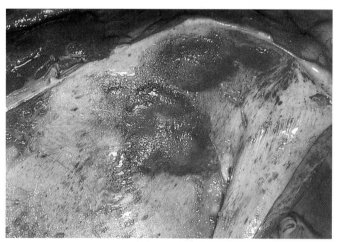

Fig. 46.1

◆ Answer 46.5
A chest radiograph should demonstrate the distribution of the pathology and this may give clues as to the type of infection. The most important investigation is the acquisition of a suitable specimen for microbiological culture; this would be sputum if the patient had a productive cough or a specimen obtained by fibreoptic flexible bronchoscopy. The nature of the infective organism and its sensitivities to antimicrobial agents is essential for accurate and efficient treatment.

◆ Answer 46.6
Fungal infections such as aspergillosis or candidiasis, *Pneumocystis carinii*, viral infections such as cytomegalovirus or measles.

◆ Answer 46.7
The function of the autopsy is not solely to determine the cause of death but to assess the extent of disease at death and its response to treatment. In this case an autopsy is important to determine the type of infection in the lungs since it may have relevance to other patients being treated on the same haematological unit.

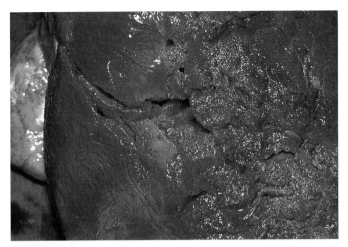

Fig. 46.2

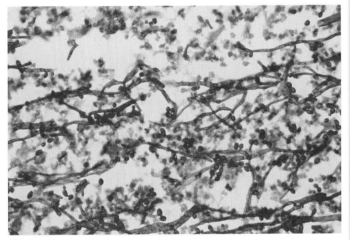

Fig. 46.3

◆ **Question 46.8**
What type of organism was causing the lung infection?

Candida is a fungal organism which is common in the environment but rarely causes infection. In this case the patient's immune defences, especially the neutrophils, were compromised by the effect of the leukaemia and the chemotherapy used to treat it and so the organism could establish itself; such infections are often called opportunistic.

◆ **Question 46.9**
Apart from leukaemias what other pathologies may predispose to opportunistic infections?

◆ **Answer 46.8**
Microscopy shows branching fungal hyphae with appearances which are consistent with *Candida* species.

◆ **Answer 46.9**
Acquired immune deficiency syndrome (AIDS) due to human immunodeficiency virus (HIV), immunosuppressive therapy associated with organ transplantation, primary immunodeficiencies due to inherited defects of the immune system such as severe combined immunodeficiency, radiotherapy, splenectomy (particularly bacterial infections), severe malnutrition and advanced cancer.

Revision

- Leukaemia, see pp. 722–728
- Autopsy, see pp. 75–76
- Opportunistic infections, see p. 216
- Pneumonia, see pp. 374–375

Pale and interesting

A 9-year-old boy of Greek parents presents at Accident and Emergency with abdominal pains, lassitude, pallor and mild jaundice. His parents speak little English and the history is difficult to extract, but it seems that he had a sprained ankle from playing football a week ago and he has had some propritary analgesics for that. He has no other significant history except his parents say he must not eat beans. The boy has not been out of the country for 5 years and no-one in the immediate family or at his school are ill. Physical examination confirms mild pallor and jaundice and there are no specific signs in the abdomen.

◆ **Question 47.1**
What tests would you do?

◆ **Answer 47.1**
Clinically he sounds as though he has anaemia and the jaundice suggests a haemolytic form of anaemia. Consequently his haemoglobin level and metabolites of haemoglobin should be determined. Jaundice occurs when serum levels of bilirubin are greater than 40 μmol/l. The bilirubin binds to connective tissue elastin and the most sensitive site for determining jaundice is the sclera of the eyes. Jaundice due to haemolysis is acholuric, that is to say there is no bilirubin in the urine but there are raised urinary levels of urobilinogen since the excess serum bilirubin is converted to urobilinogen in the gut. Reticulocytosis (reticulocytes are immature red cells that still contain polyribosomes and are capable of synthesizing haemoglobin) is also present and is a measure of the rapidity of the haemolytic process or, more strictly, the rapidity of production of new red blood cells. The haemolytic attacks destroy the older red cells first which is why early forms such as reticulocytes are found in increased numbers in the blood.

There are various mechanisms that result in haemolytic anaemia including infection, drugs, autoimmune mechanisms and various inborn errors of metabolism that result in fragility of the red cell membrane.

◆ **Question 47.2**
What is the specific test for his disease?

◆ **Question 47.3**
How does this disease differ from thalassaemia?

◆ **Answer 47.2**
In this case the most likely cause of his disease is glucose-6-phosphate dehydrogenase deficiency, Mediterranean type. Another, generally milder form, occurs in Africa. The test for this is to determine the kinetics of the enzyme glucose-6-phosphate dehydrogenase, but in practice the most common test is to determine the level of the enzyme although this has the disadvantage that some forms of the disease that might have mild alterations of the K_m alone could be missed.

◆ **Answer 47.3**
In glucose-6-phosphate dehydrogenase deficiency the haemoglobin is normal and the problems arise because of fragility of the erythrocyte membrane. Glucose-6-phosphate dehydrogenase is responsible for the production of NADPH in the cytoplasm and this is used, amongst other things, for the reduction of glutathione which in turn stabilises membranes. When the erythrocytes in these patients are exposed to infections, drugs or fava beans the membranes rupture and the contents leak out (haemolysis), which accounts for the alternative name for the disease, favism. In the thalassaemia syndromes one or other of the haemoglobin chains is either not synthesized or is produced in a smaller than normal amount and the resulting red cell abnormality causes the erythrocytes to be destroyed in the spleen. Thalassaemia is a heterogeneous collection of genetic diseases of varying degrees of clinical severity.

His progress over the next few years is unremarkable and he leaves home to attend medical school. Prior to his elective period he again consults you regarding his choice of countries in which to do his elective. He has two offers: one to go to Finland and one to sub-Saharan Africa.

◆ **Question 47.4**
Are there any problems with these?

◆ **Question 47.5**
Are there any long term consequences of this disease?

◆ **Question 47.6**
Are there any advantages in having this disease?

Revision

■ Haemolytic anaemia, see pp. 711–722

■ Jaundice, see pp. 456–457

■ G6PD deficiency, see pp. 712–713

◆ **Answer 47.4**
Visits to areas where malaria is endemic should be covered by prophylactic antimalarials and it is these drugs that are most effective in inducing haemolytic episodes in such patients. Air travel can be a problem with thalassaemic patients because of reduced oxygen levels but is not usually a specific problem for patients with glucose-6-phosphate dehydrogenase deficiency since their haemoglobin is normal.

◆ **Answer 47.5**
Long-term effects of this disease are usually related to the number of haemolytic episodes. Such patients may develop hypersplenism and pigment stones in the gallbladder.

◆ **Answer 47.6**
The abnormality of the red cell seems to confer some degree of resistance to the development of malaria, presumably because the red cells provide a less suitable environment for the parasites during their intracellular phase. It is for this reason that glucose-6-phosphate dehydrogenase deficiency has resisted elimination by natural selection since there is an opposing selection in favour of this enzyme variant that outweighs the drawbacks.

A distended abdomen

A 60-year-old woman, the wife of a general practitioner, returns from a 2-week holiday in Italy feeling less refreshed than she had expected. She has lost several pounds weight while she has been away and has not had her bowels open for 3 days. Her husband is concerned about her health and, in particular, her distended abdomen. During the night she feels nauseous and vomits.

◆ **Question 48.1**
What are the common causes of a distended abdomen?

The following morning her husband arranges for her to be seen by a surgical colleague. He visits her at home later that day and ascertains that she has no other symptoms. On examination her abdomen is distended, soft, and resonant but not tender. He performs a rectal examination: the rectum is empty; she has small haemorrhoids, but otherwise nothing abnormal is felt. A plain radiographic examination of the abdomen is performed (Fig. 48.1).

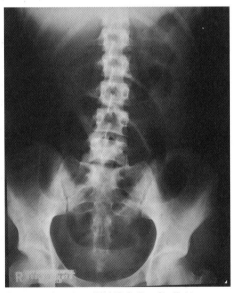

Fig. 48.1 Courtesy of Dr MC Collins, Sheffield

◆ **Question 48.2**
What is the most likely diagnosis?

◆ **Answer 48.1**
A distended abdomen is commonly due to either:

- fluid (i.e. ascites or a distended bladder)
- fat (i.e. obesity)
- fetus (i.e. pregnancy)
- faeces (i.e. constipation or obstruction)
- flatus.

◆ **Answer 48.2**
Of the various possibilities listed in answer to Question 48.1, the abdominal distension and empty rectum associated with vomiting is very suggestive of intestinal obstruction. The plain radiograph of the abdomen confirms this suspicion by revealing dilated gas-filled loops of bowel. This is a serious condition requiring urgent investigation and treatment.

The surgeon diagnoses intestinal obstruction and advises that she should be admitted to hospital.

◆ Question 48.3
What are the common causes of intestinal obstruction?

The patient's past medical history may be relevant. She has had no previous abdominal operations and no herniae are found on examination. The lack of abdominal tenderness virtually excludes peritonitis. Three years previously she had been investigated for iron deficiency anaemia. Her stools were found to contain traces of blood, and sigmoidoscopy revealed a 20-mm polyp in the sigmoid colon. The histology report reads as follows: 'This polyp is a tubulovillous adenoma showing high-grade dysplasia, but no evidence of malignancy. Excision appears complete.'

◆ Question 48.4
What connection could there be between the patient's past history and the intestinal obstruction?

The patient's condition is worsening. She has vomited a total of 900 ml of bile-stained fluid during the last 2 hours and she is feeling very weak. Blood samples are sent to the laboratory for the measurement of blood pH and electrolytes and for haematological investigations. The results are:

	Patient's values	Normal range
Sodium	145 mmol/l	143–147 mmol/l
Potassium	2.8 mmol/l	3.3–5.5 mmol/l
pH	7.4	7.35–7.45
Haemoglobin	9.0 g/dl	11.5–15.5 g/dl

The blood film is microcytic and hypochromic.

◆ Question 48.5
How do you interpret the results of these investigations?

◆ Answer 48.3
The differential diagnosis depends on the patient's age. In infants and very young children the possibilities of congenital malformations (e.g. imperforate anus), metabolic disorders (particularly cystic fibrosis) and disorders of innervation (e.g. Hirschsprung's disease) must be considered. Throughout childhood there is the possibility of intussusception. However, in this patient's age group these are the important diagnoses to consider:

- strangulated hernia
- adhesions from previous surgery
- paralytic ileus due to peritonitis
- tumours.

◆ Answer 48.4
Carcinoma of the colon is the commonest cause of large intestinal obstruction in adults, most colonic carcinomas occur in patients with tubulovillous adenomas (adenomatous polyps) and many colonic and rectal carcinomas appear to develop from adenomatous polyps. This is known as the 'adenoma — cancer' sequence. Other premalignant conditions predisposing to colonic cancer include ulcerative colitis, from which this patient does not suffer.

◆ Answer 48.5
The patient is hypokalaemic because much potassium has been lost in the vomit (intestinal secretions are rich in potassium), and the pH is high (alkalosis) because hydrogen ions have been lost with the acidic gastric secretions. The anaemia is of iron deficiency type and is most likely to be due to blood loss from a gastrointestinal ulcer or tumour.

The patient is transfused 2 units of blood and given intravenous fluid and electrolytes to restore that which has been lost. To locate the presumed obstructive lesion, a fibreoptic colonoscope is inserted though the anus. At 350 mm from the anus the colon is almost completely blocked by an annular constriction; a biopsy sample is taken, placed in 10% formalin and sent for histological examination. However, the obstruction needs to be relieved irrespective of its cause and so the patient is taken to the operating theatre where, under general anaesthesia, the abdomen is opened through a left lower paramedian incision. The colon is constricted over a length of about 30 mm by a hard mass; this is resected with approximately 150 mm colon either side and the attached mesentery. Histopathological examination of the mass reveals the appearance shown in Figure 48.2

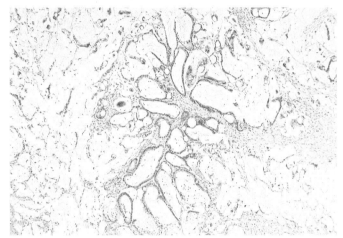

Fig. 48.2

◆ Question 48.6
What are the abnormal features?

The pathological report on the resected specimen indicates that the mass is a moderately differentiated adenocarcinoma which has invaded through the bowel wall but not metastasised to the local lymph nodes.

◆ Question 48.7
What is the Dukes' stage of this lesion and what is the likely prognosis?

Revision

- Electrolyte homeostasis, see pp. 149–150
- Adenocarcinoma of the colon, see pp. 443–444
- Staging, see p. 65

◆ Answer 48.6
This is an adenocarcinoma. The tumour is forming glands, but these are haphazard and do not have the organised arrangement seen in normal mucosa. The glands are surrounded by the smooth muscle of the bowel wall indicating that they are invasive.

◆ Answer 48.7
This is a Dukes' stage B carcinoma. Dukes' stage A tumours have invaded into but not through the bowel wall. Dukes' stage C tumours have metastasised to mesenteric lymph nodes. A Dukes' stage B carcinoma is associated with a 5-year survival rate of approximately 60%.

An itchy rash

A 35-year-old housewife who keeps several cats presents with a history of severe itching on her elbows and knees. She claims to be in good general health and a full physical examination reveals a thin but otherwise normal woman. The skin lesions are small round erosions superficial and grouped in clusters over the elbows and knees (Fig. 49.1). There is evidence of scratching.

◆ **Question 49.1**
What do you think the general type of the skin lesions might be (macules, papules, nodules, etc)?

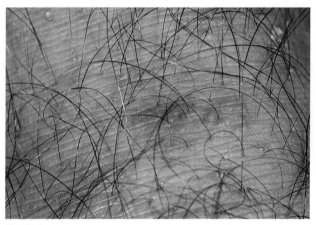

Fig. 49.1

The general practitioner identifies one small intact blister that has developed that day and excises it for histology. He sends this to the local pathology department and makes an appointment for 1 week's time.

◆ **Question 49.2**
How should the GP send the specimen to the laboratory?

◆ **Answer 49.1**
Although the skin lesions present as small superficial ulcers or erosions, further questioning reveals that they begin as small, tense blisters. They are intensely pruritic and the patient gains some relief by scratching the roof off them.

◆ **Answer 49.2**
The GP wraps it in gauze or filter paper moistened with physiological saline and sends it directly to the laboratory by messenger or taxi so that it gets there the same day. Preferably it is packed in ice. Most blistering diseases are diagnosed by a mixture of immunofluorescence (which needs fresh tissue) and routine histology (which needs fixed tissue). It is best to let the laboratory deal with this by dividing the tissue into two and processing it themselves. An early lesion with some adjacent normal skin gives the best results.

The results from the laboratory arrive:

Gross description: a 7-mm ellipse of skin with an intact 5-mm blister on the surface. Received in saline. Divided longitudinally into two; one piece fixed in formalin and the other frozen for cryostat sections.

Immunofluorescence: a band of granular IgA staining (Fig. 49.2) is seen at the intact dermo-epidermal junction. There is also linear C3 and fibrin at the junction.

Histology: there is a subepidermal blister with an inflammatory infiltrate consisting mostly of neutrophil polymorphs.

Conclusion: the appearances are diagnostic of dermatitis herpetiformis.

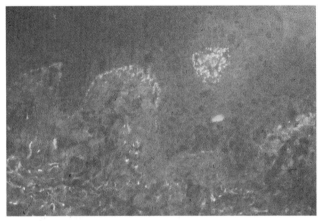

Fig. 49.2

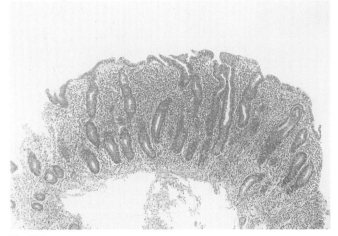

Fig. 49.3

◆ Question 49.3

What other blistering diseases are there?

◆ Answer 49.3

Intraepidermal: various pemphigus lesions.

Junctional: friction, burns, bullous pemphigoid, porphyria.

Blisters sometimes occurring with other diseases: psoriasis, eczema, lichen planus, poisons (barbiturates), drugs (both topical and systemic).

The patient defaults on follow-up but sends a letter explaining that she could not come because 'the man came to unblock the septic tank again'. She makes another appointment and her GP tells her the diagnosis and questions her carefully about the septic tank. She is embarrassed but admits to having pale, fatty faeces that smell unpleasant and are difficult to flush. They float in the septic tank and block the outflow.

◆ Question 49.4
What condition is she describing? What is it likely to be due to in her case?

You arrange for hospital investigation of her malabsorbtion.

◆ Question 49.5
What are the main causes of malabsorbtion?

◆ Question 49.6
What is the main investigation for coeliac disease?

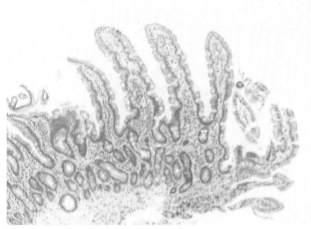

Fig. 49.4

◆ Question 49.7
Are there any long-term consequences of coeliac disease?

◆ Answer 49.4
She is describing the symptoms of steatorrhoea in which there is some malabsorbtion, particularly of fat. In her case this is most probably due to coeliac disease resulting from hypersensitivity to some component of flour, often gluten and, therefore, known as gluten enteropathy. This is frequently associated with dermatitis herpetiformis which may be the presenting complaint.

◆ Answer 49.5
Inadequate digestion: chronic pancreatitis, cystic fibrosis, bile salt deficiency
Mucosal cell disorders: gluten enteropathy, tropical sprue, Whipple's disease, giardiasis.

◆ Answer 49.6
The only certain diagnostic method involves three jejunal biopsies:

- while the patient is symptomatic which should show complete or at least partial villous atrophy (Fig. 49.3);
- following treatment with a gluten-free diet showing a significant improvement (Fig. 49.4);
- following introduction of gluten into the diet to show recurrence of the original appearances (but this is done only rarely).

◆ Answer 49.7
Overall there is a 15% increased risk of intestinal cancers, the most frequent form being small bowel lymphoma. It is not certain if good dietary gluten control affects this or not.

Revision
- Immunofluorescence, see pp. 7, 73
- Blistering disease, see pp. 765–766
- Dermatitis herpetiformis, see p. 767
- Coeliac disease, see pp. 425–427

CASE 50

A lump in the neck

A 32-year-old physical education instructor goes to see his general practitioner complaining of a lump in his neck. The patient says that the lump has been there for about 3 months and appears to have got larger. The GP examines the lump and finds it to be behind the right ear, to be 20 mm in diameter with a relatively soft texture. On further questioning the patient says that he did have an infection in the right ear earlier in the year. The doctor examines both ears with an auroscope and finds that the right eardrum is dull when compared with the left but the membrane is intact.

◆ Question 50.1
How might the lump in the neck relate to the ear infection?

The GP prescribes a course of antibiotics and asks the patient to return if the lump does not subside. Two months later the patient comes back to the surgery saying that the lump is still present, he also complains of feeling tired and of sweating at night. The GP re-examines the lump and finds that it has increased in size to 30 mm in diameter and has a rubbery firm texture.

◆ Question 50.2
Is this lump still likely to be due to a lymph node enlarged in response to infection?

The GP refers the patient to a surgeon at a local hospital who excises the lump and sends it for histopathological examination. Under the microscope at low power the lymph node has the appearances shown in Figure 50.1, and at greater magnification the appearances shown in Figure 50.2.
The histopathology report is:

Macroscopic appearances:
A firm lymph node measuring 25 × 20 × 10 mm with a pale cut surface

Microscopic appearances:
Sections show that the normal lymph node architecture has been effaced and replaced by a heterogeneous population of lymphoid cells including some large cells with single eosinophilic nucleoli and multiple nuclei. Surrounding these cells are small lymphocytes, plasma cells and some eosinophils. The areas of lymphoid cells are divided by bands of collagenous fibrous tissue

Summary:
The appearances are those of a malignant lymphoma.

◆ Answer 50.1
The lump may be a lymph node which has enlarged in response to the ear infection by hyperplasia of the lymphoid cells which have been stimulated by the infecting agent.

◆ Answer 50.2
No. Despite antibiotic therapy the lump has increased in size and now has a firm rubbery texture.

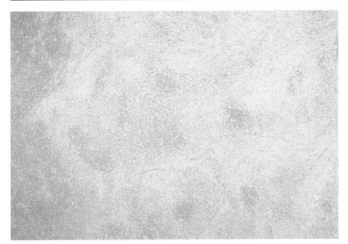

Fig. 50.1

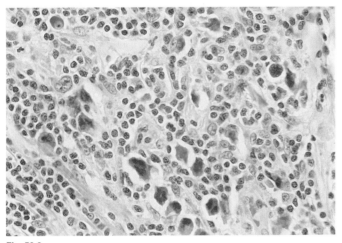

Fig. 50.2

◆ Question 50.3
What other information would you like the histopathologist to give?

◆ Question 50.4
What type of lymphoma do you think this is?

◆ Question 50.5
Can you identify which subtype of Hodgkin's disease this is (using the Rye classification)?

◆ Question 50.6
What other information about the tumour will be required before an accurate prognosis can be made and appropriate treatment selected?

◆ Question 50.7
What staging system is used in Hodgkin's disease?

◆ Answer 50.3
The pathologist has not given the type of lymphoma and such information is necessary for selection of appropriate treatment for the patient.

◆ Answer 50.4
The large cells seen in the microscopic pictures and described in the pathology report are Reed-Sternberg (RS) cells and the background of other lymphoid cells is appropriate so a diagnosis of Hodgkin's disease can be made.

◆ Answer 50.5
The bands of fibrous connective tissue and the lacunar variant RS cells which are present put this case into the nodular sclerosing category of Hodgkin's disease (the other types are lymphocyte-predominant, mixed cellularity and lymphocyte-depleted). These different categories carry different prognostic implications; lymphocyte-predominant has the best prognosis and lymphocyte-depleted the worst.

◆ Answer 50.6
The prognosis of any tumour will depend on the type of tumour (including its histological grade) and how far it has spread (its stage) so in this case assessment of the stage of the tumour needs to be made.

◆ Answer 50.7
The Ann-Arbor system (named after the place where a conference on Hodgkin's disease was held) is used. This system has four stages from I (involvement of a single lymph node region) to IV (disseminated involvement of one or more extralymphatic organs). In addition the absence or presence of systemic symptoms is shown by the suffix A or B.

◆ **Question 50.8**
Does this patient have any B symptoms?

◆ **Question 50.9**
What effect does the presence of B symptoms have on the prognosis?

Revision

■ Lymph node enlargement, see pp. 659–674

■ Lymph node biopsy, see pp. 598, 659

■ Hodgkin's disease, see pp. 663–667

■ Staging, see pp. 67, 664

◆ **Answer 50.8**
Yes, he has developed a fever. Other B symptoms are weight loss of greater than 10% and night sweats.

◆ **Answer 50.9**
The prognosis is worse with the presence of B symptoms than absence in Hodgkin's disease of a similar type and stage.

'I turned over and felt my arm crack'

A 75-year-old woman on the radiotherapy ward complains of pain in her left humerus. She says that she turned over in the night and felt her arm crack. She did not call for attention 'because the nurses were so busy'. On examination the humerus is tender and swollen at about midshaft. There is crepitus and the bone feels abnormal in that area.

◆ Question 51.1
How would you investigate this patient further?

The radiologist's report says that this patient has a pathological fracture of the midshaft of the humerus and that most other bones in her body show 'incipient fractures' (Figs 51.1 & 51.2).

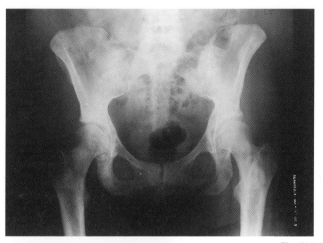

Fig. 51.1

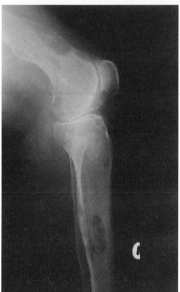

Fig. 51.2

◆ Answer 51.1
Physical examination suggests that she has a pathological fracture. This implies a fracture through abnormal bone, which seems likely from the history since you would not expect normal bone to fracture without significant trauma. Patients on radiotherapy units are likely to be on significant doses of analgesics and this patient was receiving such large doses of analgesics at home that she had been admitted for adjustment of her drugs for more effective pain control without drowsiness. Consequently her pain tolerance was quite high. She had a general set of radiographs taken in order to assess the degree of bone involvement.

It is important always to review any previous radiographs and in this patient's case there was a large collection of these. Her clinical notes also revealed that she had reported similar episodes in the past on previous admissions with similar radiograph and clinical findings.

◆ **Question 51.2**

How do you interpret this report? What is the likely cause of this patient's bone problems?

The case notes show that this patient had breast cancer 15 years ago which was treated by mastectomy and radiotherapy and that she had no further problems in the scar or in the other breast (Fig. 51.3).

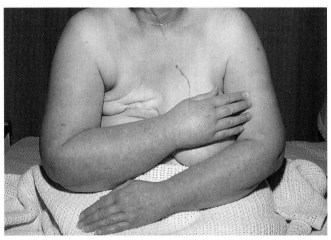

Fig. 51.3

◆ **Question 51.3**

Is it possible that her current problems are due to the old breast cancer or to the treatment that she received at that time? Are there any other possibilities?

Over the next few days the patient complains of constipation, abdominal pain and nausea. She begins to vomit, and she becomes confused and paranoid.

◆ **Question 51.4**

What are the possible reasons for this?

	Patient's values	Normal range
Calcium	3.1 mmol/l	2.02–2.60 mmol/l
Phosphate	1.8 mmol/l	0.8–1.4 mmol/l
Urea	8.4 mmol/l	2.5–6.6 mmol/l
Potassium	5.5 mmol/l	3.8–5.0 mmol/l

◆ **Answer 51.2**

This patient had multiple bone metastases which were lytic causing rarefaction of bone with increased fragility.

◆ **Answer 51.3**

It is possible for secondary deposits of primary cancers of all types to appear many years after the initial presentation, although the longer the disease-free period the more likely it is that a total cure has been achieved. New malignancies can arise at any time as they can in people without previous malignant disease, but in this lady's case no new tumour could be found and the histology of the metastatic deposits was similar to the initial breast tumour.

It is unlikely that the original treatment for breast cancer could be the cause of her current problems. It is possible to cause avascular necrosis of bone by radiotherapy but this requires massive doses and would not stay quiescent for 15 years. A late and rare complication of mastectomy with lymph node resections is lymphangiosarcoma but this presents as a massive growth of malignant tissue at the site of the original lymph node clearance extending down the arm. Some degree of lymphoedema is often present following surgery and less commonly this may persist but the malignant change to lymphangiosarcoma is very rare.

◆ **Answer 51.4**

Constipation, nausea and vomiting are frequent side-effects in patients on multiple drug therapies and this should always be borne in mind as a possibility; high doses of powerful analgesics can cause a wide range of psychiatric symptoms. In any patient with neoplastic disease, the possibility of brain secondary deposits must be considered. However, in the context of significant bone destruction, hypercalcaemia is a real possibility. Selected electrolyte values are shown in the adjacent table. Phosphate, urea and potassium are also

In the same ward there is a 16-year-old boy with a tender swelling below the right knee and a 40-year-old woman with Bence-Jones proteinuria.

◆ **Question 51.5**
What neoplasms are they likely to have?

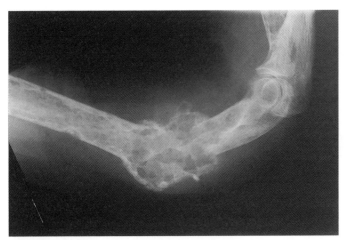

Fig. 51.4

Revision

■ Bone tumours, see pp. 798–801

■ Metastasis, see pp. 284–287

■ Multiple myeloma, see pp. 731–733, 801

■ Tumour markers, see pp. 260, 612–613

■ Hypercalcaemia, see pp. 150, 515

---

raised due to mild renal failure and dehydration. The patient was treated with active rehydration using potassium containing fluid and her serum calcium levels returned to near normal with considerable symptomatic improvement.

If untreated, calcium levels may continue to rise and at levels of 3.75 mmol/l and above there is a significant risk of death from cardiac arrest.

◆ **Answer 51.5**
Secondary tumours in young boys are very rare and this is likely to be a primary osteosarcoma. As in all cases of neoplasia it is essential to obtain a tissue diagnosis by means of biopsy and histology since the treatment is often drastic. In this case the biopsy confirmed the diagnosis and the boy had an above-knee amputation and a course of chemotherapy.

Bence-Jones proteinuria is the presence of monoclonal immunoglobulin light chains in the urine. This is characteristic of myeloma, a malignant proliferation of plasma cells (Fig. 51.4). This disease is of great historical significance because the primary structure of immunoglobulin light chains was determined using this protein; most physiological means of producing light chains at the time produced polyclonal proteins. Bence-Jones proteins are an example of an important phenomenon called tumour markers. These are substances occurring in patients indicating the presence of a neoplasm. Other examples are carcinoembryonic antigen (CEA) which may indicate the presence of intestinal malignancies and human chorionic gonadotrophin (HCG) which is produced by some malignant tumours of the placenta.

Headache

A 55-year-old male complains of headaches. He has suffered from migraine for the last 30 years, for which he has taken paracetamol, but his current symptoms are of a different character and distribution: they are frontal and throbbing.

◆ **Question 52.1**
What is the pathophysiological basis of headaches?

Worried by these new headaches, he sees his general practitioner. Routine examination includes blood pressure measurement. The systolic pressure is 180 mmHg; the diastolic pressure is 110 mmHg. Hypertension is diagnosed.

◆ **Question 52.2**
What are the main causes of hypertension?

The patient is referred to a local physician with an interest in hypertension. As part of routine investigations in new cases of hypertension, the size of the kidneys is determined by ultrasound. The pole-to-pole length of the right kidney is 60% of the left kidney.

◆ **Question 52.3**
Why could one kidney be smaller than the other?

The ultrasound investigation is followed by renal arteriography (Fig. 52.1).

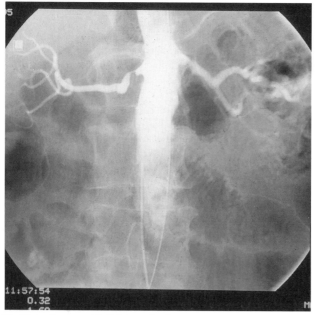

Fig. 52.1   Courtesy of Dr P Gaines, Sheffield

◆ **Answer 52.1**
There are no pain receptors in the brain itself. Although headaches may denote the presence of disease within the brain, the pain is due to irritation of pain receptors in the meninges or in the extracranial structures. Most headaches are idiopathic (without known cause), but specific causes include:

- migraine
- meningitis
- raised intracranial pressure
- temporal (giant cell) arteritis.

◆ **Answer 52.2**
Most cases of hypertension are due to unknown cause; 'idiopathic' 'essential' and 'primary' are synonyms for this common type of hypertension. Secondary hypertension may be due to:

- renal disease
- aortic coarctation
- primary adrenal neoplasms
- steroid therapy.

◆ **Answer 52.3**
Asymmetric kidneys may be due to:

- congenital maldevelopment
- unilateral ureteric obstruction causing hydronephrosis
- chronic pyelonephritis causing asymmetric scarring
- tumour affecting one kidney
- unilateral renal ischaemia.

◆ **Question 52.4**
What abnormality is revealed by the arteriogram?

◆ **Question 52.5**
What are the causes of renal artery stenosis and what is the relationship to hypertension?

A diagnosis of hypertension secondary to renal artery stenosis is made. The patient is advised to have the stenosis relieved by balloon dilatation (inserting a catheter, with a balloon at its tip, via the femoral artery into the orifice of the renal artery and inflating the balloon to stretch the orifice). This is done and, 3 weeks later, the blood pressure has fallen to 140/100 mmHg.

The patient's blood pressure remains well controlled for the next 2 years. However, he then defaults from regular follow-up.

Three years after his original presentation, the patient suddenly collapses in a restaurant. The ambulance team arrives to find him unconscious, but breathing and with a strong pulse. He is taken to the local hospital.

◆ **Question 52.6**
What is the likely explanation for his sudden collapse?

The patient is found to have a right hemiparesis and a blood pressure of 190/130 mmHg. Haemorrhages and exudates are noticed in the retinas of both eyes. A diagnosis of malignant hypertension complicated by cerebral haemorrhage is made and the patient is admitted to the hospital. The patient remains comatose for the next 3 days, but on the fourth day he responds to painful and auditory stimuli. A week later he is able to move his right arm and to speak but his speech is slurred.

◆ **Question 52.7**
How can the patient's cerebral function recover if neurones are 'permanent' cells and cannot be replaced if damaged?

After a further week, the patient develops a slight pyrexia (39°C) and, on examination, is found to have crepitations in the bases of both lungs. He is also coughing up green sputum.

◆ **Answer 52.4**
Stenosis of one renal artery.

◆ **Answer 52.5**
Renal artery stenosis may be due to either fibromuscular dysplasia or atheromatous narrowing; the latter is much more common and the likely cause in a 55-year-old male.

Renal ischaemia results in the release of renin from the juxtaglomerular apparatus. Renin activates angiotensin. Angiotensin increases arteriolar smooth muscle tone, increasing peripheral vascular resistance, and stimulates the adrenal cortical zona glomerulosa to produce aldosterone which acts on the renal tubules to enhance the reabsorption of sodium ions and water; these effects combine to increase blood pressure.

◆ **Answer 52.6**
Although sudden 'collapse' is often due to acute myocardial ischaemia, the combination of sudden onset of unconsciousness with a strong pulse suggests a non-cardiac cause. The most likely explanation is a 'stroke'. This is an important complication of hypertension.

◆ **Answer 52.7**
Although the neurones destroyed by the haemorrhage cannot be replaced, the initial loss of cerebral function was in part due to sublethal hypoxia of the adjacent neurones and oedema of the surrounding brain tissue. As the oedema and pressure subsides, so the neurones recover some function.

◆ **Question 52.8**
What complication has ensued?

The patient's condition worsens and, 3 weeks after his sudden collapse, he dies. At autopsy, the immediate cause of death is confirmed to be bronchopneumonia. There is a large resolving haematoma in the left cerebral hemisphere, consistent with cerebral haemorrhage. The heart weighs 600 g and shows left ventricular hypertrophy in response to hypertension. The aorta is severely atheromatous with tight stenosis of the right renal artery orifice. The left kidney is 200 g, the right kidney is 50 g.

Revision

■ Hypertension, see pp. 319–324

■ Renal artery stenosis, see p. 321

■ Cerebral haemorrhage, see pp. 836–837

■ Bronchopneumonia, see pp. 372–373

◆ **Answer 52.8**
The patient has probably developed bronchopneumonia, a common complication in patients with cerebrovascular accidents which often proves fatal. Indeed, if the disability from the cerebrovascular accident is very great, there may be some justification in not actively treating the infection. Furthermore, antibiotic therapy is often ineffective because the infection is due to a combination of bacteria with various sensitivities.

Blood pressure

You are a general physician with an interest in hypertension. A 39-year-old man has been referred to you by a local general practitioner who found him to have a blood pressure of 180/100 at a life-insurance medical.

◆ Question 53.1
What are the special considerations in dealing with a relatively young severely hypertensive patient?

The patient arrives and on questioning you note that he has recently been suffering from headaches, which he attributes to stress related to his company's staff appraisal scheme. He looks nervous and is pale. While taking his blood pressure, which is now 190/110, you notice that he is sweating profusely. His radial pulse is rapid at 110 per minute.

◆ Question 53.2
Are there any other pulses which you should check?

You discover that apart from the hypertension, there are no other abnormal physical signs.

◆ Question 53.3
What should your strategy be for investigating his hypertension?

Your investigations include a 24-hour urine collection for vanillylmandelic acid (VMA).

◆ Question 53.4
What is the purpose of this?

◆ Question 53.5
Are there any precautions which the patient should take while collecting his 24-hour urine sample?

The patient's 24-hour urinary VMA level comes back as more than three times the upper limit of normal.

◆ Question 53.6
What does this imply and what should you do?

◆ Answer 53.1
In general systemic hypertension is usually 'primary' (without known cause). In patients under 40, an increased proportion of cases are 'secondary' (with a known cause) and may therefore be treatable.

◆ Answer 53.2
You should check his femoral pulses to exclude coarctation of the aorta which is a cause of systemic hypertension and is usually associated with weak or delayed femoral pulses.

◆ Answer 53.3
You need to look for all the treatable causes of hypertension including the vascular, cranial, renal and endocrine causes. You also need to assess the effects that the hypertension is having on the patient by doing a chest radiograph to look for cardiac enlargement and an electrocardiogram to look for left ventricular strain.

◆ Answer 53.4
This is to look for excess excretion of VMA, which is a catecholamine metabolite increased in patients with phaeochromocytoma, for which this patient's symptoms and signs are classical.

◆ Answer 53.5
Depending on the analysis technique used by your local laboratory, the patient should avoid certain foods which can falsely elevate the urinary VMA result. You should check which these are with your local laboratory.

◆ Answer 53.6
It implies that the patient has a phaeochromocytoma. This can be located by computerised tomography scanning of the retroperitoneum and by ^{131}I-mIBG scanning.

The patient is found to have a left adrenal phaeochromocytoma (Fig. 53.1, after excision and Fig. 53.2 after slicing).

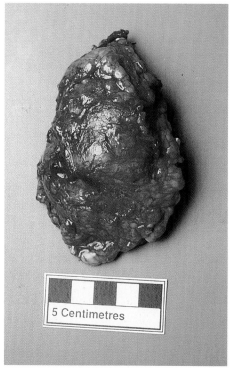

Fig. 53.1

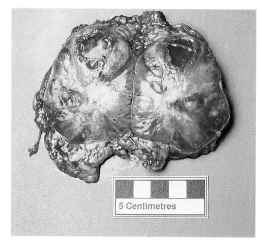

Fig. 53.2

◆ **Question 53.7**
What characteristic feature can you see in Figures 53.1 and 53.2?

◆ **Question 53.8**
Uncharacteristically, the histopathologist will not forecast the likely behaviour of the phaeochromocytoma. Why is this?

Revision

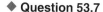

- Hypertension, see pp. 319–324

- Phaeochromocytoma, see pp. 493–494

◆ **Answer 53.7**
The tumour is brown, due to the catecholamine metabolites which it contains.

◆ **Answer 53.8**
About 10% of phaeochromocytomas pursue a malignant course but it is not possible to predict which ones will do this from the histological appearances.

'I must be allergic to something'

A patient presents to her general practitioner with a recent history of scaly lesions on the arms. She is 35 years old, and currently works as a wages clerk in a hospital although she had previously trained as a nurse. She is unmarried and has no children. She has no unusual hobbies, does a little gardening, keeps two cats and uses a wide range of cosmetics which she often changes because she has a 'sensitive skin'. On examination she has various scaly lesions of different sizes and age restricted to the extensor surfaces of the arms.

◆ Question 54.1
What are the likely causes of this skin rash?

She is given some bland cream and a mild sedative since she complains that the irritation is disturbing her sleep. She returns 2 weeks later with more lesions which have now extended to the extensor surfaces of her thighs and on to her upper chest. The GP refers her to a dermatologist. After further treatment with bland creams and antihistaminics she is given a short course of topical hydrocortisone cream. None of this is effective. A skin biopsy is performed and whilst the result of this is awaited a series of patch tests is performed.

◆ Question 54.2
What are patch tests?

The patch tests are negative except for nickel which is mildly positive.

◆ Question 54.3
What is the significance of the positive nickel patch test?

◆ Answer 54.1
Possibilities include eczema which may be idiopathic (such as atopic eczema) or caused by contact with allergens (many plants, cosmetics or chemicals in the work place) or diseases such as psoriasis.

◆ Answer 54.2
Solutions of the most common allergens are placed on the skin of the back and occluded with dressings. A range of other substances that the patient may come into contact with in their work or hobbies are often also included. After 24 hours the dressings are removed and the exposed sites are examined and any reactions are recorded then and again at 48 hours. If an eczematous or blistering rash is seen at any of the sites this is good evidence that the patient is allergic to that substance and should avoid contact with it.

◆ Answer 54.3
Nickel is a very common component in cheap jewellery and many patients are nickel sensitive to some degree, although often not enough to cause more than mild scaling beneath a wristwatch or at the site of earrings.

The histology shows non-specific chronic inflammatory changes and superficial necrosis of the epidermis.

◆ Question 54.4
What possibility will the pathologist raise in this case?

When the patient next attends she has several new lesions.

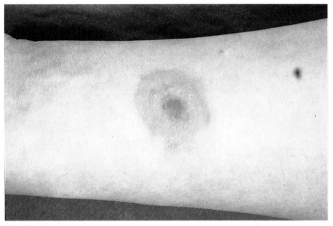

Fig. 54.1

◆ Question 54.5
What test does the dermatologist perform?

The dermatologist confronts the patient with her interpretation of the lesions and the patient becomes very aggressive and leaves, threatening legal action. She subsequently transfers to a new GP and is lost to follow-up.

Revision

- Eczema, see p. 750
- Hypersensitivity reactions, see pp. 192–204

◆ Answer 54.4
Very few diseases cause necrosis of the outer aspect of the skin without severe damage to the underlying tissue first. This suggests that the insult comes from outside and raises the possibility that the patient is causing the lesions (factitious dermatitis or dermatitis artefacta). The lesions are often bizarre in shape and distribution and, if produced by liquids, will often show drip trails (Fig. 54.1).

◆ Answer 54.5
Since the materials used to produce such lesions are often strong chemicals, wet pH paper will often show strong acid or alkali still present on the skin.

A disastrous holiday

A man of 25 presents to his GP on return from an 18–30 holiday in Spain. While he was there he had a 'flu like illness and was treated with a short course of tablets by a local doctor. The 'flu like illness resolved but two days after returning to the UK he developed a rash on his buttocks, aches and pains all over his body, mild haematuria, fever, sweating and general malaise. On questioning he admits to several sexual contacts, some without the use of condoms, and to taking illicit drugs including marijuana and ecstasy. On examination he is febrile, has a nodular, tender rash on his buttocks with scattered lesions elsewhere, he is mildly hepertensive and has a tachycardia.

◆ Question 55.1
What are the possibilites?

The GP starts the patient on a non-steroidal anti-inflammatory drug and oral corticosteroids and arranges for an urgent referral to a physician at the local hospital. At the outpatient clinic the next day the patient has become so ill he is admitted as an emergency. On the ward a number of investigations are instigated including a skin biopsy (Fig. 55.1).

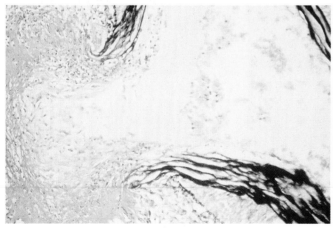

Fig. 55.1

◆ Question 55.2
What does the skin biopsy show?

◆ Answer 55.1
There are a number of possibilities from the history, including food poisoning, an allergic reaction to drugs (both prescribed and illicit drugs) and sexually communicated disease. The examination reveals a tender, nodular rash most prominent on the buttocks. This, together with the history of prescribed drugs (probably antibiotics such as sulphonamides or penicillin) for a 'flu like illness, strongly suggest a vasculitis. The rest of the history and signs and symptoms are entirely consistent with this.

◆ Answer 55.2
The skin biopsy shows a vasculitis with fibrin in the walls of vessels, chronic inflammatory cells in the walls and around vessels together with foci of thrombosis within vessels. The elastic van Gieson stain (EVG) shows dramatic rupturing of some vessel walls (Fig. 55.1).

In spite of large doses of corticosteroids the patient deteriorates over several days with worsening of renal function and some episodes of cerebrovascular events (minor fits, 'absences', confusion and mild paranoia). He suffers a cardiac dysrhythmia, arrests and cannot be resuscitated.

◆ **Question 55.3**
What autopsy findings would you anticipate?

◆ **Answer 55.3**
At autopsy there are ischaemic lesions associated with inflamed vessels and haemorrhage throughout the body including the kidney (Fig. 55.2), bowel (Fig. 55.3), and lung (Fig. 55.4) as well as in the brain and heart; this wide range of sites of vascular damage show why the presentation and the organs affected in vascular disease can be so varied and so clinically confusing. Coronary artery thrombosis is the immediate cause of death. The vessels show thrombosis due to inflammation as distinct from the thrombosis (endarteritis obliterans) which can occur in areas of general inflammation.

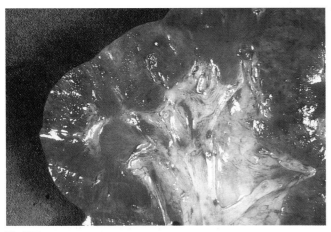

Fig. 55.2

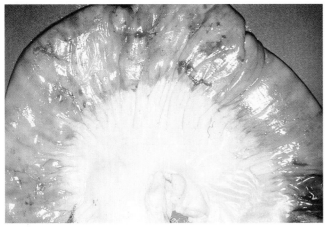

Fig. 55.3

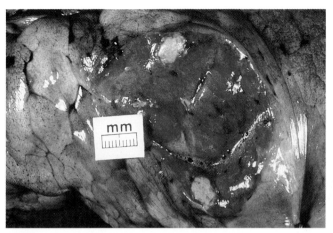

Fig. 55.4

◆ **Question 55.4**
What mechanism is responsible for the vascular injury in this case?

◆ **Question 55.5**
After the autopsy has been performed a haematology report arrives from a blood sample taken just before the patient died. It shows a mildly raised ESR. What is its significance and would it have altered treatment if it arrived earlier?

Revision

■ Vasculitis, see pp. 325–326

■ Immune complex disease, see pp. 196–198

■ Autopsy, see pp. 75–76

◆ **Answer 55.4**
The mechanism of this kind of reaction is usually due to immune complex deposition in vessel walls with subsequent inflammatory destruction. Consequently episodes of ischaemia can often be followed by episodes of haemorrhage as the vessels first thrombose and are then destroyed. The clinical picture of vasculitis depends upon the type of vessels involved. The pattern described here of involvement of muscular arteries associated with a probable drug reaction and haemorrhage from vessels is characteristic of polyarteritis nodosa. However, there is considerable overlap in the vasculitides and it is often impossible to assign a specific name to a given clinical case.

◆ **Answer 55.5**
A raised ESR is a very non-specific finding that occurs in a great variety of clinical situations and only indicates that the patient is ill. Of itself it demands no treatment; one should always treat the patient, not laboratory results.

Skin rash and arthritis

A 20-year-old athletic female student presents at routine fol-low-up after a recent appendicectomy. She is well, the wound has healed and the stitches have been removed but she com-ments that the scar is 'flaking'. On examination there is a silvery, scaly lesion following the line of the scar. The patient says that if she scratches the scale it bleeds in little points.

◆ **Question 56.1**
What is the skin rash?

◆ **Question 56.2**
What are the two eponymous signs described here?

◆ **Question 56.3**
Are the appearances diagnostic?

On closer questioning the patient also describes a history of 'dry skin' on the elbows. In the family history the father had died in a road traffic accident soon after the patient's birth but is said to have had a skin problem and severe finger-nail abnormalities.

A skin biopsy of her rash would have the appearances seen in Figure 56.1.

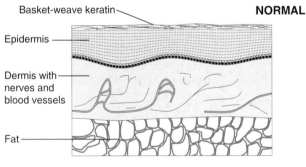

NORMAL

Basket-weave keratin

Epidermis

Dermis with nerves and blood vessels

Fat

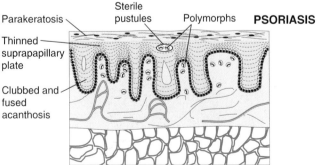

PSORIASIS

Sterile pustules

Parakeratosis

Polymorphs

Thinned suprapapillary plate

Clubbed and fused acanthosis

Fig. 56.1

◆ **Answer 56.1**
Psoriasis is a common skin condition (about 2% of the population). It is a chronic skin disease with numerous associated conditions (or it is a systemic disease in which the skin manifestations dominate). It is inherited, probably as an autosomal dominant condition, but the exact mode is not clear as penetrance and expression seem to vary.

◆ **Answer 56.2**
Psoriasis often develops at sites of trauma and it may present in this way as it did here; this is known as the Koebner phenomenon. Several other skin diseases show this phenomenon including viral warts and lichen planus.
  In psoriasis the epidermis is very disordered with greatly thickened rete ridges and very thinned epidermis between the rete ridges (above the dermal papillae) this results in pin-point bleeding when the patients scratch the lesions and this is called Auspitz's sign.

◆ **Answer 56.3**
The combination of clinical features is so characteristic that most dermatologists would not need a biopsy to confirm the diagnosis. When a biopsy is taken the histological appearances seen in Figure 56.1 are diagnostic: there are nuclear fragments in the keratin (parakeratosis); the epidermis is thickened (acanthosis); the epidermis is thin over the dermal papillae; there is a neutrophil infiltrate in the dermis and entering the epidermis.

Thirty years later the patient is being seen for joint pains in the hands and feet and a stiff neck. She is apyrexial and her blood picture and blood chemistry are normal. Rheumatoid factor is negative. Figure 56.2 shows foot radiographs. Figure 56.3 shows a photograph of her hands. She now has an extensive skin rash, most severe over extensor surfaces (Fig. 56.4).

Fig. 56.2
A

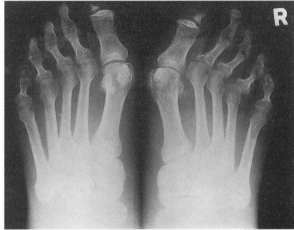

B

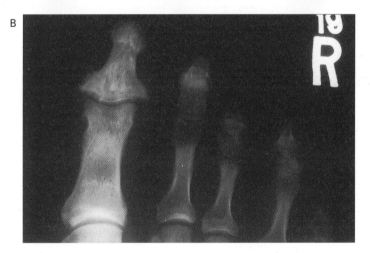

Fig. 56.3

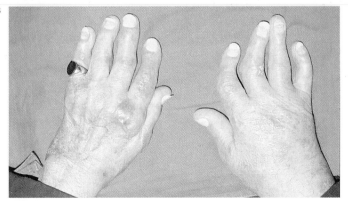

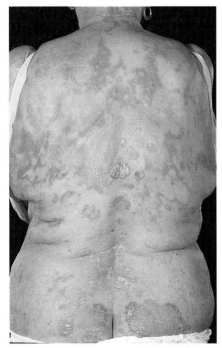 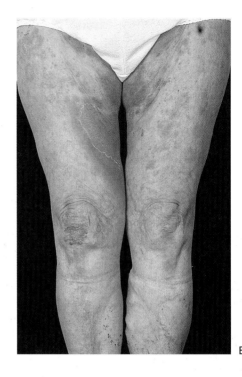

A

B

Fig. 56.4

◆ Question 56.4

What abnormalities are there in the radiograph? Why may she have a stiff neck?

Revision

■ Psoriasis, see pp. 758–759

■ Psoriatic arthropathy, see p. 812

◆ Answer 56.4

The clinical picture of the hand shows the destructive arthropathy. The foot radiograph (Fig. 56.2) show a highly desructive arthropathy affecting terminal interphalangeal joints preferentially. Psoriatic arthropathy is a relatively late complication but is quite common. A rather more rare but still very characteristic complication is ankylosing spondylitis in which vertebrae, commonly in the neck, fuse.

CASE 57

Swelling in the neck

A 55-year-old woman has been referred to your surgical out-patients clinic by a local general practitioner. She is troubled by a swelling in her neck which has been slowly getting larger.

She comes into your consulting room and you take a history. She has lived in Derbyshire all her life, has had no major illnesses and is asymptomatic apart from having noticed a swelling in her neck. She is having no trouble swallowing or breathing. Her neck is shown in Figure 57.1.

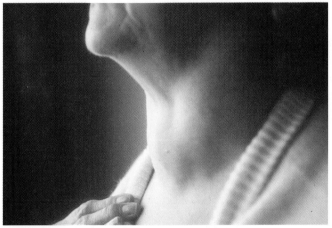

Fig. 57.1

◆ Question 57.1
How can you determine from what neck structure the mass in Figure 57.1 originates, by physical examination?

You discover that the patient's thyroid feels enlarged and has a mass approximately 25 mm in diameter in the right lobe.

◆ Question 57.2
What is the differential diagnosis of a thyroid mass?

You send off the patient's thyroid function tests and perform fine-needle aspiration cytology of the apparent thyroid mass. The mass disappears after aspiration.

◆ Question 57.3
What does this tell you about the mass?

◆ Answer 57.1
You should sit the patient down, give her a glass of water and palpate her neck from behind while asking her to swallow. If the mass is, or originates from, the thyroid, it will move down with swallowing.

◆ Answer 57.2
This includes colloid cysts and nodules in a multinodular goitre, benign neoplasms (for practical purposes the only one is follicular adenoma) and malignant neoplasms (of which there are several types).

◆ Answer 57.3
It indicates that the mass was really a cyst.

You arrange for the patient to have an ultrasound examination of the thyroid gland and to come back in 2 weeks' time.

◆ Question 57.4
What can ultrasound tell you about the thyroid gland?

The patient returns in 2 weeks' time. Her thyroid function tests are within normal limits. The ultrasound examination revealed a multinodular goitre.

◆ Question 57.5
What is the aetiology of multinodular goitre?

You have already seen the fine-needle aspirate at your weekly case conference with the pathologist. It looked like Figure 57.2.

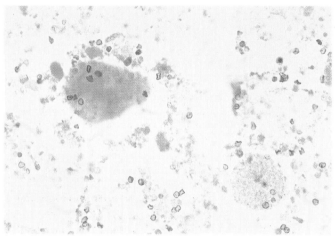

Fig. 57.2

◆ Question 57.6
What does Figure 57.2 show?

You discuss the findings with the patient. She is not keen to undergo surgery, especially as the goitre is not causing any symptoms. You discharge her from follow-up having reassured her, but advise her to come back if she has any further problems.

2 years later you are giving a dinner party when at 23.30 your registrar telephones you. The patient has been sent in to hospital by her general practitioner with a 2-hour history of discomfort in her neck and difficulty in breathing.

Because you are the consultant on call you have not been drinking so you drive to the hospital where you discover that the patient is in moderate respiratory distress due to a new 40 mm mass in her right thyroid lobe.

◆ Question 57.7
What is likely to have happened?

◆ Answer 57.4
It can reveal residual masses after aspiration and show up whether the rest of the thyroid is normal or whether there is in fact multinodular goitre.

◆ Answer 57.5
It is relative underproduction of thyroxine by the thyroid leading to a compensatory increase in thyroid stimulating hormone secretion by the pituitary. This leads to episodes of focal hyperplasia in the thyroid which eventually lead to a gland consisting of many nodules separated by fibrous tissue. Dietary lack of iodine, which occurs in Derbyshire, can cause the initial underproduction of thyroxine.

◆ Answer 57.6
It shows proteinaceous fluid consistent with colloid and a few foamy macrophages, telling you that the lesion was a colloid cyst.

◆ Answer 57.7
The acuteness of the history suggests that the patient has haemorrhaged into a cyst in the multinodular goitre.

You operate to remove the multinodular goitre. The resected specimen is shown in Figure 57.3.

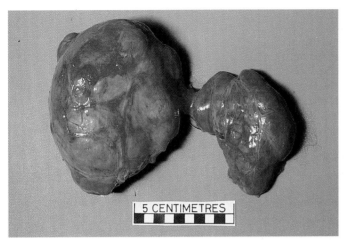

Fig. 57.3

◆ **Question 57.8**
What can you see in Figure 57.3?

You resist the temptation to cut into the thyroid mass and submit the gland whole for histophathological examination.

◆ **Question 57.9**
Why should you not cut into excised lesions?

The histopathology report comes back indicating a multi-nodular goitre with recent haemorrhage into a cyst. The patient makes an uneventful recovery and is eventually discharged home on regular thyroxine replacement.

◆ **Answer 57.8**
The gland shows overall multinodularity and there is a mass in the right lobe.

◆ **Answer 57.9**
All masses may be malignant tumours. The histopathologist needs to assess completeness of excision. If you cut into the tissues, you create a false apparent resection margin which can lead to completely excised lesions appearing to be incompletely excised.

Revision

■ Thyroid disease, see pp. 502–508

■ Cytopathology, see pp. 68–70

■ Histopathology, see pp. 5, 65, 71–72

A tinctorial diagnosis

A 58-year-old man presents to his general practitioner complaining of swelling of his legs and breathlessness whilst walking up hills. He is a lifelong smoker of cigarettes and on questioning it is found that his diet contains a high proportion of saturated fat. He has had rheumatoid arthritis for many years and has received non-steroidal anti-inflammatory drugs (NSAIDS), steroids during acute exacerbations and one course of gold injections. On examination there is pitting oedema of both legs and crackles at the bases of both lungs.

◆ **Question 58.1**
What is the likely cause of the patient's symptoms?

The GP takes a blood sample and sends it to the clinical chemistry department of the local hospital. The results come back:

	Patient's result	Normal range
Sodium	136 mmol/l	130–147 mmol/l
Potassium	4.3 mmol/l	3.3–5.5 mmol/l
Urea	10.2 mmol/l	3.3–8.3 mmol/l
Creatinine	230 μmol/l	60–120 μmol/l
Calcium	2.23 mmol/l	2.12–2.63 mmol/l

◆ **Question 58.2**
What do these values show?

◆ **Question 58.3**
What might be causing renal failure in this patient?

The patient is given pharmacological therapy for his heart failure but his condition continues to deteriorate and he dies during a brief hospital admission. The clinicians obtain permission from the relatives for a hospital consent autopsy. At autopsy the spleen has the appearance shown in Figure 58.1 and the heart, after the application of Lugol's iodine has the appearance shown in Figure 58.2. Histological sections of the heart, stained with Congo red dye, have the appearances shown in Figure 58.3 which changes to the appearances shown in Figure 58.4 when viewed with polarised light:

◆ **Answer 58.1**
The patient has the signs and symptoms of heart failure.

◆ **Answer 58.2**
These results are compatible with a moderate degree of renal failure.

◆ **Answer 58.3**
In patients with a degree of cardiac and renal failure it is often difficult to sort out which came first. In marked heart failure the kidneys will be underperfused and there will be secondary renal failure, in renal failure there may be fluid retention and secondary heart failure. This patient could have ischaemic heart disease due to coronary artery atherosclerosis (with risk factors of cigarette smoking and a high saturated fat intake) with secondary renal failure. Alternatively he could have renal failure from a variety of different causes, such as a membranous glomerulopathy associated with gold therapy or immune complex glomerulonephritis, and secondary cardiac failure.

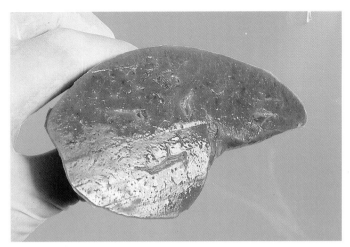

Fig. 58.1

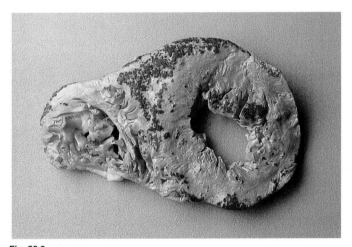

Fig. 58.2

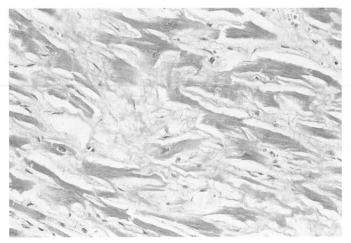

Fig. 58.3

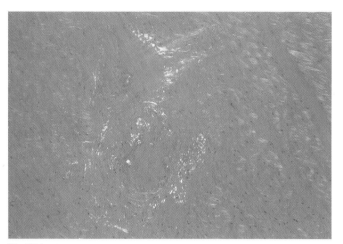

Fig. 58.4

◆ **Question 58.4**
What is the cause of this patient's heart failure?

◆ **Question 58.5**
What sort of amyloid is this likely to be?

◆ **Question 58.6**
What other types of amyloid are there?

◆ **Question 58.7**
What is the characteristic structure of amyloid protein?

Revision

■ Renal function impairment, see pp. 90, 335, 590, 628, 816

■ Amyloid, see p. 388

■ Rheumatoid arthritis, see pp. 805–811

◆ **Answer 58.4**
Systemic amyloid deposition including deposition in the myocardial cells with resultant impairment of contractile function. The deposited amyloid protein stains brown with Lugol's iodine at macroscopic examination, red with Congo red and produces an apple-green dichroism when viewed with polarised light after Congo red staining. The spleen has a 'glassy' macroscopic appearance due to amyloid deposition.

◆ **Answer 58.5**
It is likely to be a reactive amyloidosis (with AA protein) associated with the patient's rheumatoid arthritis.

◆ **Answer 58.6**
Myeloma-associated, senile, haemodialysis-associated, hereditary and familial (neuropathic, familial Mediterranean fever) and local amyloid in endocrine tumours (such as medullary carcinoma of the thyroid).

◆ **Answer 58.7**
A beta-pleated sheet.

A fatal delivery

A 25-year-old previously fit prima gravida undergoes an uneventful delivery of a healthy child. The next day she collapses with severe respiratory distress, cyanosis and cardiovascular shock.

◆ **Question 59.1**
What is shock?

In spite of active treatment she begins to fit and rapidly lapses into deep coma.

◆ **Question 59.2**
What is the most likely cause of this collapse?

Within two hours she shows signs of severe pulmonary oedema and begins to bleed from the birth canal. The various laboratory findings are shown in the following table.

	Normal range	Patient's values
Prothrombin time (seconds)	21	11–14
Activated partial thromboplastin time (seconds)	70	30–40
Thrombin clotting time (seconds)	19	10–12
Plasma fibrinogen (g/l)	0.8	2.0–3.0
Platelets (10^9/l)	20	150–400
Serum fibrin degradation products (μg/ml)	128	<8
Fragmented red blood cells in peripheral film	many	none

◆ **Answer 59.1**
Shock is circulatory collapse and represents a mixture of the pathological effects of low circulatory volume relative to the vascular volume and the physiological attempts to overcome this. Shock can be the result of various pathological insult: loss of blood volume due to haemorrhage, burns, vomiting, diarrhoea (hypovolaemic shock); increase in vascular volume due to infection (septic shock); loss of effective circulatory volume due to myocardial infarction, dysrhythmia, pulmonary embolus (cardiogenic shock). Other more obscure causes include retained products of conception in the uterine os during incomplete abortion and amniotic fluid embolism (sometimes called amniotic infusion in the USA). The physiological responses to these conditions involve adrenergic activation causing peripheral vascular shut down directing blood to vital areas, tachycardia and incidental sweating. This leaves the patient cold, clammy, cyanosed and hypotensive with a thready pulse. Volume replacement and treatment of the underlying cause are the basis of therapy.

◆ **Answer 59.2**
This is a classic presentation of amniotic fluid embolus. A tear in the placenta during labour allows amniotic fluid into the maternal circulation, helped by the high pressures developed within the uterine cavity during labour. The amount of amniotic fluid detectable in the lungs is commonly too small to explain the devastating clinical condition and it is assumed that chemical factors, such as prostaglandins and tissue thromboplastins contained within amniotic fluid, may precipitate pulmonary vasoconstriction and impaired cardiac contractility.

◆ **Question 59.3**

What has happened now?

Her clotting parameters swing wildly out of control and, in spite of active therapeutic intervention, the patient dies with signs of hepatic and renal failure.

◆ **Question 59.4**

What post mortem findings would your anticipate?

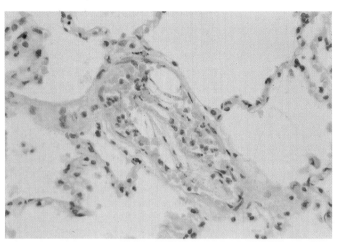

Fig. 59.1

Revision

■ Shock, see pp. 178–180

■ Blood coagulation, see p. 691

■ Disseminated intravascular coagulation, see pp. 740–742

■ Pathology of pregnancy, see pp. 576–584

■ Amniotic fluid embolism, see p. 379

◆ **Answer 59.3**

In those cases where rapid, spontaneous resolution does not occur then the next phase is disseminated intravascular coagulation (DIC). This has also been called consumption coagulopathy as rapid sequences of thrombosis and alternating haemorrhage occur, eventually using up (consuming) the various substances involved in thrombosis and thrombolysis.

From the table it is obvious that the measurements of time taken for various clotting processes are all much increased (prothrombin time, activated partial thromboplastin time and thrombin clotting time) indicating that bleeding will be much more prolonged than in a normal subject. The substances in the blood concerned with clotting are depleted (plasma fibrinogen and platelets) and the breakdown products of clots (fibrin degradation products) are much increased showing that clots are forming and being destroyed at a great rate. The fibrin meshworks that are being produced in small vessels hamper the free passage of red cells and damage them giving rise to increased numbers of fragmented red cells.

DIC as a result of amniotic fluid embolus is commonly fatal.

◆ **Answer 59.4**

At autopsy, skin squames from the baby were found in the lung vasculature (Fig. 59.1) and widespread signs of both haemorrhage and thrombosis were found in most tissues.

A visit to Australia

A 60-year-old woman, who has just returned to the UK from visiting her married daughter in Australia, attends her GP complaining of felling 'off colour'. She takes little exercise due to her weight and disposition, has numerous aches and pains and is mildly breathless; she is voluble and says that she ate all sorts of foreign food and was bitten by numerous insects in Australia. On examination she is moderately obese, apyrexial, in normal sinus rhythm and complains of tenderness in various sites, including both claves. There are faint respiratory crackles in the lung fields but no specific signs. The GP prescribes low dose aspirin.

◆ **Question 60.1**
Is this placebo treatment in order to get rid of a tiresome patient?

Two days later the patient's husband calls the GP out in the early morning. The patient is now acutely short of breath and very tender over one calf which is swollen and inflamed. The patient is pale and cyanosed with cold extremities.

◆ **Question 60.2**
What is the likely sequence of events here?

Stasis

◆ **Answer 60.1**
No. The GP intends this as rational treatment since he suspects that a possible cause of the patient's symptoms is a venous thrombosis in the calf with small fragments breaking off to cause mild episodes of breathlessness. But, although aspirin reduces clotting, it is only effective in arterial clots such as coronary artery thrombosis. There is no evidence that aspirin reduces the risks from deep vein thrombosis or the related propagation of the thrombus which can lead to pulmonary embolism. The proper treatment is effective anticoagulation with heparin and with warfarin (both of which inhibit clotting) which needs careful monitoring of clotting capacity.

◆ **Answer 60.2**
It is likely that the immobility of a long plane flight from Australia could result in relative immobility of the legs with an increased risk of thrombus formation, particularly in the legs in an obese subject. Drinking alcohol on the flight could also lead to some degree of dehydration and a tendency to increased risk of thrombosis. The small thrombi in the calf veins are not a great problem and will generally resolve with normal activity, but further thrombus can be deposited upstream from the initial thrombus and as this gets into larger veins, such as the femoral or iliacs, the chances of it breaking off and embolising become greater. The chances of such large emboli causing clinical problems are also much greater. The factors that predispose to thrombosis are: changes in the vessel wall; changes in the flow of blood; changes in the nature of the blood. The first of these is more important in arterial thrombi and the other two are most important in venous thrombosis. These three factors are collectively known as

◆ **Question 60.3**
What should the GP do?

On admission to hospital the patient is assessed and an ECG is performed which shows elevated waves in S1, Q3 and T3 as well as 'right heart strain'.

leads?

◆ **Question 60.4**
What does this ECG report mean?

◆ **Question 60.5**
What is the appropriate treatment?

As she is being prepared for treatment the patient has a cardiac arrest and, in spite of active resuscitation attempts, she dies.

Virchow's triad and any one or combination of them predisposes to thrombosis; it does not need all three.

◆ **Answer 60.3**
The GP arranges emergency admission to hospital having diagnosed probable massive pulmonary embolism.

◆ **Answer 60.4**
This is the classical picture of massive pulmonary embolism also known as acute right-sided heart failure. ?

◆ **Answer 60.5**
Anticoagulation will prevent further episodes but the acute treatment would be to introduce thrombolytic agents, such as urokinase, intravenously onto the clot via a long intravenous catheter. Introduction of such agents elsewhere into the peripheral circulation does not get adequate amounts to the site of the embolus.

◆ **Question 60.6**
Should this case be reported to the coroner?

◆ **Question 60.7**
What might you expect to find at autopsy?

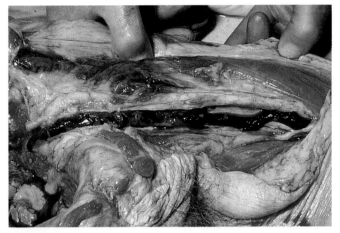

Fig. 60.1

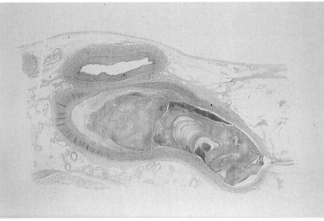

Fig. 60.2

◆ **Answer 60.6**
Because the GP has seen the patient
within the last few days and both he and
the casualty officer are certain of the
cause of death there is no statutory
reason to report this case to the coroner.
However, in most localities there is a
convention to report all deaths occurring
within 24 hours of hospital admission
since this covers the great majority of
cases that might fall under the coroner's
jurisdiction and provides a safety net for
doubtful cases. The coroner does not
take the case and the casualty
department has a policy of asking for
relative's consent for post mortems on
all patients who die under their care. The
relatives agree but stipulate that the
head must not be opened. The relatives
have a right to stipulate such limitations
and these are legally binding in consent
(so-called 'hospital') autopsies; they may
not make such stipulations in coroner's
cases. The post mortem is carried out
that day, which is policy in the pathology
department in order not to delay funeral
arrangements.   *Counsel?*

◆ **Answer 60.7**
The post mortem reveals residual
thrombus in the calf veins (Fig. 60.1)
which is confirmed on histology
Fig. 60.2) and massive pulmonary
embolism in the main pulmonary arteries
(Fig. 60.3) with focal lung infarction
(Fig. 60.4).

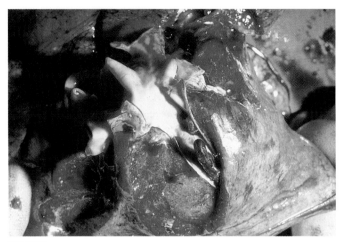

Fig. 60.3

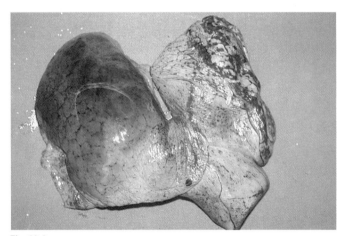

Fig. 60.4

Revision

■ Thrombosis, see pp. 166–169

■ Pulmonary embolism, see pp. 169–171, 379

■ Medicolegal autopsies, see pp. 75, 399

Index to presentation

Note: The index refers to CASE rather than page number

Index to diagnosis (possible, differential and definitive)
Note: The index refers to CASE rather than page number

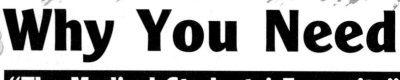

Why You Need

"The Medical Students' Favourite"

General and Systematic

Pathology

Edited by JAMES C E UNDERWOOD

2nd Edition

Paperback   948 pages   250 line, 30 h/t, 370 colour illus   July 1996   0 443 05282 4

"The medical students' favourite"; a full colour textbook of pathology for undergraduate medical students. Targeted directly at the core syllabus, **General and Systematic Pathology** provides the essential information you require, and presents pathology in the context of modern medicine and cellular biology.

Your First Choice in Pathology
- Logical structure for ease of use
- High-quality colour diagrams and illustrations throughout
- Style is thorough, but not overdetailed
- Highlighted key points and summaries convey core facts easily
- Detailed glossary of pathological terms
- Outlines and explains disease mechanisms

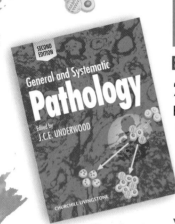

Contents

PART 1
BASIC PATHOLOGY: Introduction to pathology / characteristics, classification and incidence of disease / genetic and environmental basis of disease / pathology in clinical practice.

PART 2
DISEASE MECHANISMS: Disorders of growth, differentiation and morphogenesis / responses to cellular injury / metabolic and degenerative disorders / thrombosis, embolism and infarction / immunology and immunopathology / inflammation / carcinogenesis and tumours / ageing and death.

PART 3
SYSTEMATIC PATHOLOGY: Cardiovascular system / respiratory tract / alimentary system / liver, biliary system and exocrine pancreas / endocrine system / breast / female genital tract / male genital tract / kidneys and urinary tract / lymph nodes, thymus and spleen / blood and bone marrow / skin / bones, joints and connective tissues / central and peripheral nervous systems.

Also available as an
INTERNATIONAL STUDENT EDITION IN ELIGIBLE COUNTRIES

REVIEWS
of the first edition

"Most students would find the text easy to read and informative. They will be helped greatly by the excellent illustrations of gross pathology, good diagrams and helpful lists and tables."

Histopathology

"There was no doubting the medical students' favourite – Underwood. I mentioned it to my tutorial group one week; by the next session most had a copy; by the end of term over half the year had a copy; and by the beginning of the next term all the tutors had a copy."

Journal of Pathology

"I would unreservedly recommend this book as the basis from which to revise for the pathology exams for the vast majority of students."

Guy's Hospital Gazette

Customer Services
Freephone (UK only): 0500 556 242
Phone: +44 (0)131 535 1021   Fax: +44 (0)131 535 1022

CHURCHILL LIVINGSTONE   Robert Stevenson House, 1–3 Baxter's Place, Leith Walk, Edinburgh EH1 3AF, UK